PARKINSON'S DISEASE

A Guide for Patient and Family

Du Pont is pleased to present you with this copy of
"Parkinson's Disease:
A Guide for Patient and Family"
by Roger C. Duvoisin, M.D.

As is the case with most publications, this book
does not include complete information about
indications, contraindications, warnings,
precautions, adverse reactions, and dosage for
the drugs discussed. Therefore, we ask you to
refer to the enclosed Prescribing Information for
SINEMET® (Carbidopa-Levidopa) before
prescribing.

The opinions and recommendations expressed
in this book are those of the author and
do not necessarily reflect the opinions and
recommendations of Du Pont.

Pharmaceuticals and Imaging Agents

Parkinson's Disease

A Guide for Patient and Family

Second Edition

Roger C. Duvoisin, M.D.

Professor of Neurology and Chairman, Department of Neurology
The University of Medicine and Dentistry of New Jersey
Robert Wood Johnson Medical School

Chief, Neurology Service
Robert Wood Johnson University Hospital
New Brunswick, New Jersey

Raven Press 🖑 New York

Raven Press, 1185 Avenue of the Americas, New York, New York 10036

Made in the United States of America

Library of Congress Cataloging in Publication Data

Duvoisin, Roger C.
  Parkinson's disease.

  Includes bibliographical references and index.
  1. Parkinsonism. I. Title. [DNLM: 1. Parkinson
disease—Popular works.   WL 359 D987p]
RC382.D94   1984   616.8′33   83-13714
ISBN 0-89004-904-1
9

Preface to the Second Edition

The warm and generous reception accorded the first edition of this book, in its several printings, is gratefully acknowledged. It provided reassuring vindication of that undertaking, and showed that the trepidation I had felt on first writing the book was fortunately unfounded. It also confirmed my feeling that there was a need for a simple straightforward presentation of the essential facts about parkinsonism.

It seems difficult to believe that 5 years have passed since the book first appeared in print. Yet in those years, substantial advances have been achieved in our understanding of parkinsonism, or rather, of the parkinsonisms. New concepts of treatment have evolved. New drugs have been introduced. Perhaps as a result of the dramatic rise of local support groups, the wide dissemination of information by the newsletters of the various Parkinson Foundations, and the generally more open discussions of chronic disorders in the public media, patients and their families have become more knowledgeable about their disorder. They are eager to keep abreast of the latest developments. To meet their needs and interests I have revised the text, expanding some sections to cover new topics such as brain transplantation and sexual dysfunction, and adding a chapter on the dopaminergic receptor agonists. I have been greatly aided in this effort by the many readers who have sent helpful comments and criticisms. To them and to my patients I express my thanks.

Roger C. Duvoisin

Preface to the First Edition

Appreciable advances have taken place during the past 10 to 15 years in our understanding of the nature of parkinsonism and more specifically of Parkinson's disease. Treatment has become much more effective but also more complicated. Consequently, the success of treatment depends more than ever on the cooperation of the patient and the family. The best cooperation is built on intelligent understanding of the disease process itself, of what the doctor is trying to do, and of how the treatment actually works. But, alas! There is too little time in the daily bustle and rush of medical practice to explain all that needs explaining and to answer all the questions asked by every patient. Then too, patients often think of the most important questions after they have left the doctor's office, and forget them by the time of the next visit. Some questions are difficult to ask, and perhaps the patient does not know how or what to ask. It is often preferable and easier to find the answers in private, in a book.

Many pamphlets and monographs have been offered to the Parkinson patient over the years with a view to explaining the symptoms or providing a system of exercises or a method of treatment. Many of these are excellent, but most are out of date, and few have attempted to provide a comprehensive account. Patients often complain of the saccharin quality of much of this material. One of my older patients, after reading an especially benign review, growled that its author had "made the disease sound like it was a pleasure to have." Like most patients, this fellow did not want an inspirational message or psychotherapy. He wanted and needed a simple, forthright account about what was going on in his body, what could be done about it, and how to do it. The late Dr. Lewis Doshay's popular monograph *Parkinson's Disease: Its Meaning and Management* served this purpose when it was written nearly 20 years ago. Subsequently, however, the treatment of parkinsonism has been radically changed by the development and availability of levodopa and then by the enzyme-inhibitor drugs carbidopa and bensarizide. The surgical treatment of parkinsonism has been largely abandoned. Newer forms of treatment undreamed of when Dr. Doshay wrote his book are even now under clinical study. Thus there seems to be a genuine need for an up-to-date book on the subject addressed to patients and their families in adequately detailed but nontechnical terms.

I have tried to answer this need in the present volume and to give the lay reader a comprehensive account of current concepts of the basic nature of Parkinson's disease and other forms of parkinsonism, some understanding of its treatment, and explanations of its more common symptoms. I have done this in essentially the same manner in which I discuss these subjects with patients and their families in the privacy of my office.

It was not without some trepidation that I set out on this task for I was uncertain of the wisdom of dealing with all the major and many of the minor symptoms of Parkinson's disease in a single volume. So numerous and varied are the symptoms that few patients experience them all. I feared that it would be impossible to avoid telling more about the disease than the reader would care to know or perhaps should know. Patients with a particular set of symptoms might be dismayed to learn of still others they had not yet experienced and perhaps never would. In short, I was worried that the burden of full knowledge might be too great for some to bear. Such, after all, was the concept of the physician's responsibility to the patient taught to the medical profession over the past century and persuasively stated by the great physician-teacher Sir William Osler in his essay entitled *Equanimitas*.

The past quarter-century, however, has seen important changes in these stern old Victorian attitudes toward sickness and health. Patients now want to know all they can about their diseases, and we recognize their right to complete access to the medical truth. We no longer need to write our prescriptions in Latin so that the patients may not know what medicines they are taking. The fear that patients may not be prepared by training and experience to accept the truth has not been vindicated. The new openness has proved in many ways to be unexpectedly healthy. It is obvious in practice that patients fare better and can face their problems with equanimity and intelligence when they gain a reasonable understanding of their affliction, of what their doctor is trying to do for them, and of what can be done with treatments currently available.

Thus I have tried to present a plain, unvarnished account of Parkinson's disease and other forms of parkinsonism, realistically describing the nature of the disease, the various symptoms, the side effects (as well as the good effects) of current drug therapies, and the limits of our present knowledge. In the blunt language of our time, I have tried to "tell it like it is." I must add one word of explanation: In describing the signs and symptoms, I relied on my observations of patients made before the advent of levodopa. The efficacy of this drug is such that many of these manifestations are now quite rare or, when they do occur, are relatively mild. Nevertheless I thought it important to present as complete a picture as possible.

Because I believe that patients with chronic disorders who must take medication for indefinite periods should know what drugs they are taking, why they are taking them, and what the side effects are, I devoted a large part of this book to describing the various drugs used in treating parkinsonism. In describing the drugs, I used the generic names and indicated the trademark names in parentheses. When several trade names exist, I indicated the one which is most familiar or most commonly used. I do not mean thereby to recommend one product over another. The generic equivalent drugs are, to my knowledge, indistinguishable in their effects and serve equally well. I mentioned the trade names employed in the United States and Canada. The same drugs are available in most countries but sometimes under different proprietary (trade) names.

To a limited extent I ventured into the scientific knowledge underlying the present concepts of parkinsonism. Because these concepts are not fixed but are in constant flux, I thought it important as well as interesting to try to put our present concepts and knowledge in some historical perspective. I also tried to share with the reader the hopes of research and prospects for still better treatment in the years ahead.

Much of the material in this volume has been presented in various lectures I have given over the years to patient groups, nurses, physical therapists, social workers, and lay audiences. To a very considerable extent this book reflects the many things I have learned from my patients and their families. I humbly acknowledge the great debt I owe them for all they have taught me, not only about their disease but about themselves as people, about life itself, of courage in the face of long adversity, and of the remarkable strength of the human spirit. I trust that I have been able to convey what I have learned from them to others who may benefit from this collective experience.

Finally I wish to acknowledge the encouragement of Dr. Alan Edelson, my publisher, the able editorial assistance of Virginia Martin and Laura Kosden of Raven Press, the helpful criticism of my son Marc, whose journalist's eye caught many a syntactical error, and of my friends Charles and Rhoda Kaufman.

Roger C. Duvoisin

Contents

PARKINSON'S DISEASE

A Guide for Patient and Family

CHAPTER 1

What Is Parkinsonism?

The word parkinsonism refers not to a particular disease but to a commonly recognized condition marked by a characteristic set of symptoms. Chief among these are trembling of the limbs, muscular stiffness, and slowness of bodily movement. To this triad may be added a tendency to stand in a stooped posture; to walk with short, shuffling steps; and to speak softly in a rapid, even tone.

The trembling usually affects the hands and feet but sometimes also the lips, tongue, jaw, abdomen, and chest. It tends to occur in the affected hand or foot when it is at rest and to disappear during a movement. For example, trembling in the hand ceases while reaching out to pick up an object but reappears when the hand is returned to a position of rest. The trembling, or *tremor*, is thus a *resting tremor*, unlike tremors in other disorders.

The muscular stiffness is also of a particular kind. It is called a "plastic *rigidity*" because a doctor examining an affected person finds a constant, uniform resistance to passive manipulation of the limbs. The affected muscles seem unable to relax and are in a state of contraction even at rest.

The third element of the triad, the slowness of bodily movement, is called *bradykinesia* (from the Greek *brady*, meaning slow, and *kinesis*, meaning movement). It is a very complex phenomenon comprising hesitancy in initiating a new movement or activity, slowness in its execution, and rapid fatiguing. The term bradykinesia also encompasses a lack of spontaneity and a diminution in the performance of the automatic movements of which we are usually unaware, such as eye blinking, the swing of the arms while walking, expressive gestures of the hands while talking, facial expressive movements, etc.

THE UNDERLYING DYSFUNCTION

This complex of symptoms we call parkinsonism reflects the dysfunction of a particular region of the brain—in fact, of a particular system of nerve cells in a center or nucleus known as the *substantia nigra*. It is called the substantia nigra, a Latin expression meaning "black substance," because it is deeply pigmented and may readily be seen by the naked eye on examining specimens of human brain (Fig. 1). It can be seen under the microscope that the dark color of the substantia nigra is due to pigment granules densely packed within

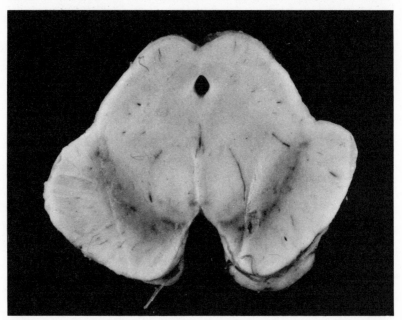

FIG. 1. Specimen of human brain cut transversely through the upper brain-stem to show the substantia nigra. This is the appearance in a normal brain.

the nerve cells that reside in that nucleus. This pigment seems to be chemically similar to the melanin pigment responsible for the color of our skin and eyes, and so it has been called neuromelanin. We do not know its chemical structure precisely nor what its function may be. However, we believe that this pigment is related in some way to the fact that these nerve cells produce and store a specific chemical substance called *dopamine*. Similar pigment granules are also found in other nerve cells, mainly in cells which produce and store dopamine and the closely related substances adrenaline[1] and noradrenaline.

The nerve cells of the substantia nigra send long, thin fibers upward to connect with other nerve cells in the deep gray matter of the cerebral hemispheres known as the *corpus striatum* (Fig. 2), or *striate body*. Dopamine made in the cells of the substantia nigra travels up these fibers to the corpus striatum, there to act as a chemical messenger transmitting signals to the nerve cells of the striatum. When the substantia nigra cells are injured or for some reason cannot produce or store dopamine, there results a deficiency of dopamine in the striatum. If the deficiency is sufficiently severe, symptoms of parkinsonism begin to appear. Some neuroscientists have defined parkinsonism in chemical terms as a state of brain dopamine depletion.

A deficiency of brain dopamine can come about in various ways. The nerve cells of the substantia nigra may deteriorate for one reason or another. They may be injured by a tumor, a stroke, a chemical agent, or a virus infecting the brain (encephalitis). Brain dopamine deficiency can also be caused by certain drugs. A functionally comparable state can be caused by drugs which block the action of dopamine in the striatum. The dopamine is then unable to deliver its chemical message, and the end result is the same as when dopamine is deficient. Similarly, if the nerve cells of the striatum which normally receive the chemical messenger dopamine lose their ability to receive the message, the effect is the same as when do-

---

[1]Adrenaline is the common name for this substance. Scientists frequently refer to it as epinephrine. Adrenaline and epinephrine are one and the same.

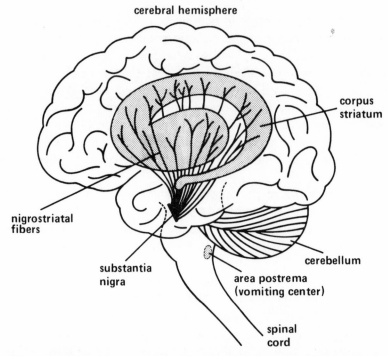

FIG. 2. Left side view of the human brain showing schematically the substantia nigra and the corpus striatum *(shaded area)* lying deep within the cerebral hemisphere. For simplicity, only one side is shown. Nerve fibers extend upward from the substantia nigra and, dividing into many branches, carry dopamine to all regions of the corpus striatum.

pamine is absent. This is believed to be the situation in certain disorders. Without going into further detail, it is clear that there are many possible causes of parkinsonism, some more important than others and some very rare.

PARKINSON'S DISEASE

By far the most prevalent type of parkinsonism today is the condition first described by James Parkinson in 1817 in his *Essay on the Shaking Palsy*. It is generally known as Parkinson's disease. It was the first type of parkinsonism to be recognized and remains the prototype against which other types are compared. It is sometimes called *idiopathic* parkinsonism or *paralysis agitans*. The term idiopathic means that the cause is unknown. Paralysis agitans is merely "shaking palsy" translated into Latin; it is the official name for the disease in the World Health Organization's International Statistical Classification of Disease.

The cause of Parkinson's disease is not known. Pathologists classify it as a *system* degeneration of the brain because specific groups or systems of nerve cells appear to be the target of some morbid process. The disease process seems to select very precisely only certain nerve cell systems. It is clearly not a random thing. The location of the affected cells is such that their deterioration almost certainly cannot be due to poor circulation or to arteriosclerosis. Nor is there any sign of infection or inflammation. The selective involvement of certain systems of nerve cells scattered through the brain and spinal cord suggests that an unknown toxin or a deficiency of some undiscovered nutrient may be responsible. Some think that there is merely a premature aging process which affects the cells of the substantia nigra. The truth is that the cause or causes are simply unknown.

The disease rarely affects people under the age of 40 years. The average age of onset seems to be about 60 to 61 years. The beginning is usually so insidious and the progression so gradual that it can rarely be dated precisely. Usually the first symptoms noted are, to quote James Parkinson, "a slight sense of weakness, with a proneness to trembling . . . in one of the hands and arms." These symptoms tend to increase very gradually year by year over a period of many years. Indeed, progression is so gradual that little if any changes can be seen from one year to the next.

Parkinson's disease is believed to affect about a half-million persons in the United States, or approximately 1% of the population over age 50. It occurs with a similar prevalence in other countries in which good epidemiological studies have been done and appears in all races of mankind all over the world. It is difficult to make precise comparisons in different countries, however, owing to differences in medical care systems and in statistical methods. Some statistical data are available in England and Wales dating back to the middle of the last century and from various hospitals and university clinics in the United States and several European countries at least as far back as the 1890s. These data suggest that the prevalence of the disease has not changed appreciably over the past century.

There is a widespread suspicion that Parkinson's disease is genetically determined. Many patients ask whether their disease is hereditary or runs in families. It is true that approximately 10 to 15% of patients report that they have an affected relative. However, when one actually examines these relatives, it turns out that many—more than half in my experience—have some other disorder. The remaining relatives who do in fact also have Parkinson's disease do not represent a greater number than would be expected by chance. After all, if everyone has at least ten relatives who have lived beyond age 50, and the prevalence of the disease is 1% of the population over age 50, no fewer than 10 patients in a 100 would be expected to have an affected relative by chance alone.

Only rarely will Parkinson's disease affect both members of a pair of identical twins. Over the past several years, I conducted a careful study of Parkinson patients, who were identical twins, with Doctors Donald Calne, John Nutt, Roswell Eldridge, Andrew Williams, and Christopher Ward. We uncovered only 2 concordant twin pairs among 43 pairs of identical twins. That is, only 2 of 43 co-twins also had Parkinson's disease. This is strong evidence that Parkinson's disease does not have a genetic cause. There is also no evidence that the offspring of a patient with Parkinson's disease are at greater risk of developing the disease later in life than anyone else.

Occasionally one encounters a husband and wife who both have the disease, but the incidence of conjugal parkinsonism is less than 2%, approximately what might be expected by chance alone. This is good evidence that the disease is not contagious. Moreover, since it may be presumed that husbands and wives have shared a similar diet and environment for many years before the usual onset of parkinsonism, this observation is also additional evidence that a dietary factor is not likely to be the cause of the disease.

No difference in the incidence of the disease in men versus women has been found. Nor have studies of its incidence in different occupations or socioeconomic groups revealed any special concentration of cases. Parkinson's disease appears to be a democratic disease. The possibility that a virus may be involved in causing Parkinson's disease has long been an attractive hypothesis. It seems even more attractive now that the twin study has ruled out heredity as a causative factor. It has been suggested that an unconventional or incomplete virus causing a "slow" viral disease might be responsible. However, thus far, no evidence for a virus has been found.

In summary, the cause of Parkinson's disease remains a profound mystery.

DRUG-INDUCED PARKINSONISM

Another common cause of parkinsonism today is the drug treatment of mental illness such as schizophrenia. There may be as many cases of drug-induced parkinsonism as there are cases of Parkinson's disease; however, they are almost entirely found among psychiatric patients. The powerful tranquilizing drugs used in treating mental illness block the actions of dopamine in the brain. The resulting disturbance of brain function is essentially the same as that caused by depletion of brain dopamine. The great value of these drugs is that they can tranquilize without causing sedation—that is, without making the patient feel drowsy, groggy, or sleepy. Introduced into medical practice during the mid-1950s, these drugs revolutionized the treatment of mental illness. They quickly displaced the padded cell, straitjackets, water therapy, and the various coma therapies such as insulin coma, which had previously been the main methods of treatment available. However, these drugs also cause a Parkinson-like state which closely mimics Parkinson's disease and sometimes also presents features of postencephalitic parkinsonism. Efforts to find an effective major tranquilizer that does not cause parkinsonism have thus far failed. It appears that the tendency of these drugs to cause parkinsonism is linked in some fundamental way to their effectiveness in treating mental illness. Indeed, some psychiatrists believe that producing a very mild degree of parkinsonism is necessary to obtain good results in their patients. It has been said, partly in jest but with more than a grain of truth, that treatment with the major tranquilizers represents a sort of "chemical straitjacket" more humane and more effective than the old physical methods.

The first of the major tranquilizers and probably still the most familiar is the drug chlorpromazine. Its proprietary name in the United States is Thorazine and in Europe, Largactil. Many derivatives of chlorpromazine have been made and are widely used as tranquilizers. These include Stelazine, Permitil, Mellaril, and Prolixin, to cite a few of those in more common use by their trade names. One drug of this class, prochlorperazine (Compazine), is used mainly to combat nausea and vomiting. These drugs are known collectively as the phenothiazines.

A closely related chemical family includes the drug haloperidol (Haldol). This is one of the most potent of the major tranquilizers. It can induce a Parkinson-like state within 10 minutes of its injection into a vein!

One of the first tranquilizers found capable of causing parkinsonism was the drug reserpine derived originally from the Indian snakeroot plant *Rauwolfia serpentina*. It is commonly used today to treat high blood pressure. Although in large doses it can induce a state of parkinsonism, it very rarely does so in the small doses in which it is used to lower the blood pressure in hypertensive patients. Reserpine also causes a condition in animals which resembles parkinsonism, and it has consequently been used in experimental work to help find new treatments for human parkinsonism. Another drug used in treating hypertension, methyldopa (Aldomet), also, although very rarely, can produce a chemical parkinsonism. Both these drugs induce parkinsonism by causing a depletion of brain dopamine through chemical means. Several other agents are known that also induce a chemical parkinsonism, but they have been used only as experimental drugs and are not given in ordinary medical practice.

All of these forms of drug-induced parkinsonism are reversible. The Parkinson-like state they cause gradually disappears when the patient stops taking them or if the dose is simply lowered. It may take several days or perhaps 1 to 2 weeks for the parkinsonism to subside. Rarely, it takes more than a month, but parkinsonism persisting indefinitely after treatment with any drug has not been reported.

POSTENCEPHALITIC PARKINSONISM

Encephalitis means literally "brain inflammation." In common medical usage it refers to brain inflammation due to a virus infection. Parkinsonism occurring as a sequel to a viral infection of the brain is called postencephalitic, meaning that it came "post" or after the encephalitis. There is only one kind of encephalitis known to have resulted in chronic progressive parkinsonism. This was a rather unusual type of encephalitis that occurred primarily during the years 1916–1926 in small epidemics scattered throughout the world. A few sporadic cases were seen during the 1930s and the early 1940s but none since then. The first cases were seen in central Europe in 1915 and 1916, and were studied and described by the Austrian neurologist Constantine von Economo. The condition was thus widely known as von Economo's encephalitis. Because it occurred chiefly in small epidemics, it was more generally called *epidemic encephalitis*. It was also called *encephalitis lethargica* because its first symptom was prolonged sleepiness. It was popularly known during the 1920s as *sleeping sickness*—not to be confused with the sleeping sickness of central Africa transmitted by the bite of the tsetse fly.

In addition to sleepiness, the patients developed various types of strabismus, difficulty in swallowing, and bizarre changes in personality and behavior. Many patients, as many as 40 to 50%, died during the acute, or initial, phase of the illness. The survivors gradually recovered after 6 months or more, with various residual symptoms. Some remained severely crippled, with paralysis, tremors, severe muscle rigidity, marked mental changes, and many other difficulties. Some appeared to have fully recovered but later gradually began to develop such difficulties. This delayed progressive phase of the illness was called *chronic encephalitis* and later *post-encephalitis*. Eventually it became apparent that the patients had many symptoms similar to those of Parkinson's disease, and at that point they were said to have *postencephalitic parkinsonism*. Nearly all the survivors sooner or later developed this peculiar kind of parkinsonism; approximately 80% did so within 3 years of the first symptoms. The remainder were often thought to have fully re-covered, but it was later realized that they too were left with subtle residual symptoms. They were said to be "neurasthenic." They looked normal on examination, but their behavior was changed. They remained generally withdrawn and were not able to resume the pattern of their former lives and to return to school or work. They tired easily, had little initiative, and seemed generally passive. Gradually these survivors also developed some manifestations of parkinsonism, although these were sometimes very minimal. Thus eventually all the survivors developed some degree of parkinsonism. They also had many sequelae of their encephalitis that had never been seen in parkinsonian patients before. One of the most re-markable was the repeated occurrence of "visual spells" in which the head and eyes were turned up as if to look at the ceiling for hours at a time. These episodes were called "oculogyric crises." Other unusual sequelae were compulsive tics and rituals which could be so severe as to render otherwise normal-appearing persons in-capable of ordinary employment.

Although the first epidemics of encephalitis lethargica were ob-served in Europe several years before the great worldwide flu pan-demic of the winter of 1918–1919, there was nevertheless a common tendency to connect postencephalitic parkinsonism with the flu. The connection was a vague one, and many other diseases such as mul-tiple sclerosis were also thought by some to occur as a result of the flu. They were thought to be part of the "epidemic constitution" of the flu—whatever that may have meant. Since the infectious agent of the flu was not identified until 1933, it is perhaps understandable that the whole subject was confused and that many illnesses of unknown cause were suspected of being related to the great flu pandemic. No conclusive evidence has ever been found that encephalitis lethargica was a consequence of the flu.

Repeated attempts were made to isolate an infectious virus from persons afflicted with this condition, but its cause was never found. Various viruses were recovered, notably the virus herpes simplex, which we now know to be responsible for the ordinary "cold sore." Initially this virus was thought to be the probable cause, and a vaccine was prepared from it to treat cases of encephalitis lethargica. After many years of research and much effort, a great deal was learned about herpes simplex although it seemed less and less likely to be the cause of encephalitis lethargica. Looking back at the efforts of the early "microbe hunters" to find the infectious agent of encephalitis lethargica, one can only admire how much was accomplished with tools which by present standards may be called primitive. Clearly, the science of virology was not sufficiently advanced at the time to accomplish the task.

There were a great many patients with this type of parkinsonism during the 1920s and through the 1940s. In fact, postencephalitic parkinsonism was by far the commonest cause of parkinsonism seen by physicians during those years. However, very few, if any, fresh cases of postencephalitic parkinsonism have been observed during the past half century, and so it has become a very rare condition. Physicians today see only a very few oldtimers who are survivors of the epidemics of the 1920s and 1930s.

No other type of encephalitis has been found to cause anything like the sequelae of encephalitis lethargica. Some symptoms reminiscent of Parkinson's disease are seen rarely during the acute or initial phase of various kinds of encephalitis, but these nearly always disappear during convalescence and never return. Very rarely a few symptoms, such as tremor in one hand, may persist after recovery from some types of encephalitis (Japanese B encephalitis and Central European tic-borne encephalitis), but these are mild and do not progress over the years as was the case in survivors of encephalitis lethargica. Several types of viral encephalitis occur regularly in North America, usually in small, scattered epidemics. These include eastern equine encephalitis, western equine encephalitis, and St.

Louis encephalitis. They occur during the summer or early fall and are caused by a virus transmitted to humans and horses by mosquito bite. The viruses responsible for more common illnesses such as measles, chickenpox, "shingles" (herpes zoster), and the common cold sore (herpes simplex) may also on rare occasion infect the brain and produce encephalitis.

Although all these viruses have been suspected at one time or another of being responsible for some cases of parkinsonism—even for parkinsonism developing many years later—there is no factual evidence to support these suspicions; and that is not for lack of trying. Many studies have been carried out in search of some association between parkinsonism and these viruses, so far with consistently negative results. An example is the long-term follow-up surveys of survivors of western equine encephalitis carried out over a period of many years by the California Encephalitis Commission. Several cases of Parkinson's disease were found—in approximately the number that would have been expected by chance, however. Thus none of the viruses prevalent today that are capable of producing encephalitis give rise to parkinsonism or Parkinson's disease.

More recently, extensive studies of antibodies in the blood of Parkinson patients have been carried out. The presence of antibodies to a specific virus indicates that the person in question, has at some previous time, been infected by that virus. Over 30 common viruses were studied, including several strains of flu virus. No evidence was found to implicate any of the viruses studied.

ARTERIOSCLEROTIC PARKINSONISM

Elderly persons who have recovered from several minor strokes may be left with some stiffness and slowness, a tendency to walk with short, shuffling steps, and some difficulty speaking clearly. If to these symptoms is added the gently stooped posture common among the elderly, there may be a resemblance to Parkinson's disease. The resemblance is just that, a similarity in appearance. Such persons are often said to have arteriosclerotic parkinsonism. There is some argument among experts whether the term is justified because the symptoms merely resemble those of Parkinson's disease but are in fact different. The term was originally coined over 50 years ago by a prominent British neurologist, Dr. MacDonald Critchley. He has since stated he would rename the condition arteriosclerotic *pseudo*parkinsonism. In any case, it is a different disorder; and arteriosclerosis, or hardening of the arteries as it is popularly called, does not cause true Parkinson's disease. Usually there is little difficulty distinguishing between the two conditions. However, sometimes even the experts disagree. Of course, everyone over 50 years of age has some degree of arteriosclerosis, and it is always possible to have Parkinson's disease plus some brain dysfunction due to arteriosclerosis to complicate the situation. Arteriosclerotic changes are not uncommon in patients over age 70.

The differentiation of Parkinson's disease from arteriosclerotic parkinsonism is not just an academic exercise; it has some practical value in prognosticating the response to treatment. The symptoms of the latter do not respond to treatment as well as do those of true Parkinson's disease, and the elderly arteriosclerotic patients are more apt to experience side effects of drug treatment.

SYMPTOMATIC PARKINSONISM

A variety of diseases and intoxications can involve the substantia nigra, damage its nerve fibers on their long path to the corpus striatum, or injure the corpus striatum itself and thus cause some degree of parkinsonism. In such cases the parkinsonism is considered to be a symptom of another disease. For example, brain tumors may rarely, if they happen to be in the right place, result in some parkinsonian symptoms. Similarly, head injuries, congenital malformations, and various infections (such as tuberculosis or syphilis) on rare occasions cause some degree of parkinsonism.

Certain types of poisoning tend to injure selectively the corpus striatum and may cause some symptoms resembling those of parkinsonism. The best known disorders of this type are carbon monoxide poisoning, and carbon disulfide and manganese intoxication.

The damage to the nervous system caused by these substances is extensive and the symptoms are quite different from those of parkinsonism. Manganese intoxication occurs chiefly in workers mining manganese ore.

The "punch drunk" state in oldtime boxers who suffered repeated blows to the head has also been likened in some particulars to Parkinson's disease. There is also a case on record of a man who suffered a bullet wound of the brain which destroyed the substantia nigra on one side. Symptoms similar to those of Parkinson's disease developed on the other side of the body and persisted for many years without further progression.

Rarely, parkinsonism occurs in adolescents or young adults (juvenile parkinsonism) as an expression of rare hereditary disorders such as Wilson's disease, an inborn error of copper metabolism in which there is a form of copper poisoning.

PARKINSONISM PLUS

In many chronic progressive disorders of the nervous system Parkinson symptoms may occur along with some other symptoms reflecting dysfunction of the cerebellum or other parts of the nervous system. I often speak of these conditions as "parkinsonism plus." The "plus" refers to symptoms that do not occur in true Parkinson's disease. These are clearly different diseases. Their causation is essentially unknown except that some may occur in certain families, and thus are the result of a genetic or inherited factor. One group of these disorers is termed "olivopontocerebellar atrophy" (OPCA). The term merely describes the pattern of atrophy or shrinkage that may be found on anatomical examination of the brain. Another disease is termed "striatonigral degeneration." Another is the "Shy-Drager" syndrome, a rare disorder in which regulation of blood pressure, control of the urinary bladder, and sexual function are impaired. Finally, there is the rare disease named "progressive supranuclear palsy" or the Steele-Richardson-Olszewski syndrome distinguished by a disturbance in eye movements.

Collectively, these disorders are known to neurologists as the "multiple system atrophies." They account for nearly 20% of all cases of parkinsonism seen in medical practice today. They are often very difficult to distinguish from Parkinson's disease in the 1st or 2nd year of symptoms. The last three conditions were not recognized as distinct disorders until the 1960s!

Recently, a deficiency of the enzyme glutamate dehydrogenase was found in some patients with OPCA. At the time of writing, about 25 patients with this abnormality have been identified. Most had been initially diagnosed as cases of "parkinsonism." The enzyme deficiency is inherited, but may or may not give rise to symptoms within a normal lifetime. In several patients, the first symptoms developed after age 75. The full meaning of this new discovery is not yet clear, but it raises hope of a means of treatment and prevention. Testing for the enzyme should be done in new cases of parkinsonism, particularly in those with atypical features.

SUMMARY

Parkinson's disease has been known for over 150 years. It is almost certainly a specific disease, although its cause is not yet known. In addition there are many disorders which resemble Parkinson's disease in varying degrees. In some, the cause is known. There is also the remarkable fact that the major tranquilizing drugs can produce a condition that closely resembles Parkinson's disease, but disappears when the drugs are discontinued.

All these conditions resembling Parkinson's disease are called parkinsonism. Thus there is a postencephalitic parkinsonism, drug-induced parkinsonism, arteriosclerotic parkinsonism, etc. Most of these forms of parkinsonism share one thing in common with Parkinson's disease: A particular set of nerve cells in a center called the substantia nigra are injured or impaired, with the result that the brain is depleted of a chemical substance known as dopamine.

CHAPTER 2

The First Symptoms

So gradual and insidious is the onset of Parkinson's disease that patients can rarely pinpoint the precise date it began. At best, they remember when they first became aware of its presence. In many cases the first signs of the disorder appear long before the patient suspects that anything is amiss. Sometimes one can find evidence that the disorder may have begun several or even many years before its symptoms are recognized. For example, several times I have found on reviewing old home movies that a patient failed to swing one arm while walking 5 or 6 years before tremor appeared in that arm. Old snapshots may show that the patient began to have a stooped posture many years before anything was suspected.

One of my patients had once consulted a speech therapist because of a "mumbling" speech that made his work as a salesman difficult. Eight years later he developed tremor in one hand and consulted a neurologist. Tremor of the hand accompanied by rigidity of the arm as well as a soft, "mumbly" speech were noted on examination. It was then clear that the "mumbly" speech had in fact been the first manifestation of Parkinson's disease in that patient, but no one suspected the correct diagnosis until the tremor appeared. It is unlikely that even the most observant diagnostician could have found sufficient evidence to make the diagnosis when "mumbly" speech was the only problem.

Strangely, it often happens that the first sign of parkinsonism is noted not by the patient but by someone else. Usually it is someone close to the patient—a spouse, relative, friend, or colleague at work—who notices some change. Perhaps there has been a subtle change in posture or a new habit: holding one arm bent at the elbow and close to the body while walking, or stiffness of one leg when walking. The patient usually denies that anything is the matter when asked about these things. A colleague may ask: "Is anything wrong with your leg, you seem to be limping?" Or the patient's spouse repeatedly says: "Stand up straight, you're always bent over lately." Friends and family are often surprised that the patient seems unaware of these changes in posture or manner of walking or moving. They may prevail upon the patient to see a doctor. The interview in the doctor's office may go something like this:

Doctor: "Well, what brings you in today?"

Patient: "Nothing, really."

Doctor: "Nothing?"

Patient: "I feel perfectly well. There's nothing the matter with me."

The patient's spouse may then intervene to describe the cause of her concern: "Doctor, there's something wrong with his left leg when he walks."

So the doctor examines the way the patient walks. He may readily recognize the problem, but it often happens that the trouble is not apparent at the moment. Spouses often complain that the patient always looks much better in the doctor's office: "Doctor, if only you could see him when he is at home."

Most likely the doctor sees that something is indeed amiss; but the telltale signs of parkinsonism are usually not yet present at this stage of the disease, and the doctor probably cannot make the diagnosis. Perhaps he orders a few tests: a blood count, some blood chemistries, an electrocardiogram, and x-ray of the chest, and a routine analysis of the urine. This battery of tests constituting the usual "checkup" probably gives normal results. Parkinson patients seem to be a pretty healthy lot, generally speaking, an observation made by many physicians. The experienced doctor probably wants to see the patient again in a month or two or if further problems arise. At this juncture, a little "tincture of time," to quote an old medical aphorism, is appropriate. If something really is going on, it shows itself more clearly in due course.

Eventually, the patient becomes aware that something is indeed wrong. There may be persistent tiredness, minor aches and pains, or a vague sense of malaise, of just not feeling well. Perhaps the patient feels a lack of energy or a sense of nervousness and irritability. Performance on the job may be declining for no apparent reason. The patient may notice that things which were formerly done easily, without a thought, now require conscious effort. On seeing the patient again and listening to these vague complaints, the doctor can sense that there is a problem even though all the tests done at the previous checkup were normal. He may try to reassure the patient that the tests were all normal. He may urge the patient to get some rest, perhaps take a vacation, and maintain a good diet. He may even prescribe a mild tranquilizer. If the patient seems depressed, the doctor may prescribe treatment with an antidepressant drug and suggest referral to a psychiatrist. Proper treatment of depression usually helps considerably, and so the patient can carry on as usual for some time.

This phase of Parkinson's disease, in which vague, nonspecific symptoms develop, may continue for a long time. Some patients, understandably distressed by symptoms no one seems able to explain, tend to visit many doctors and clinics in search of an explanation, but the diagnosis is extremely difficult to establish at this point in the evolution of Parkinson's disease. The symptoms do not point to any specific condition. Overwork, lack of sleep, nervousness, depression, arthritis, poor dietary habits, and similar problems are more likely causes of such complaints.

Later, the patient may begin to experience more-specific symptoms, such as soreness in one arm, a sense of weakness or "numbness" in one hand, stiffness in one leg, trouble in carrying out some movement, a change in the quality of the voice. There are almost as many initial symptoms as there are patients. Each individual experiences the disorder differently and interprets the experience in his or her own way. Although these more-specific complaints indicate to the doctor that something is definitely wrong, there may still be no physical signs to suggest the nature of the problem. Even if the doctor sees something such as a tendency to "drag" one foot slightly on walking, a change in facial expression, or a tendency to "favor" one hand, he is still unable to diagnose Parkinson's disease. A single finding is not enough to establish the diagnosis, and there is no blood test (or any other kind of test for that matter) that can establish the diagnosis.

The diagnosis can be made with certainty only when the three characteristic signs are present: *tremor, rigidity,* and *bradykinesia.* Tremor is usually the first to appear. Initially it may be minimal. It may be noticed only when the patient is fatigued or under some stress. Some patients feel the tremor for many months before it is visible. If the writing hand is affected, it is common for the tremor to be noted in the patient's handwriting. Every letter tends to show evidence of a very fine tremor. Usually the handwriting is also somewhat small, a phenomenon called *micrographia.* In addition, the patient's writing tends to get progressively smaller on the page or even within a paragraph. The doctor may thus ask for a sample of the patient's handwriting to look for these signs. Occasionally tremor appears initially in a foot, and rarely in the lips, tongue, or jaw.

In a small but significant percentage of patients there is little or no tremor. Rigidity and bradykinesia may then be the first symptoms. The patient may experience only a sense of weakness of a hand or leg. There may be difficulty with fine tasks, such as buttoning up a shirt or tying shoelaces. Patients whose work or hobbies require some degree of manual dexterity may become aware of a loss of ability. In the patients who do not have tremor, the diagnosis is more difficult to establish and may not be made until relatively late in the course of their illness.

As soon as one of the three characteristic signs is evident, the doctor recognizes that there is some disturbance in the nervous system; and especially if there is tremor, he should suspect parkinsonism. Depending on the symptoms, the findings on examination, and the patient's age and general health, the diagnosis of Parkinson's disease may now be evident at a glance. However, often it is not so obvious at first, and many other possibilities cross the doctor's mind.

In many cases the symptoms concentrate on one side of the body. The patient, for example, may complain of weakness of the left arm and leg, and the doctor may have noted some evidence of such weakness on his examination. In appearance, the patient with such symptoms—walking with some loss of left arm swing and tending to shuffle with the left foot—somewhat resembles a person who has had a mild stroke.

It happens occasionally that patients convey an erroneous impression that their symptoms came on suddenly. One of my patients, for example, told me that he had first noted trouble with his right arm and leg a month previously, and that he was now somewhat better. He believed that he had experienced a stroke. However, his wife described a more gradual and remote onset of his difficulties. It seems that the trouble with the left arm and leg had been present for at least a year or more. On further questioning, it became clear that what the patient meant was that the trouble had become important enough for him to pay attention to it about a month previously, and that he had not been fully aware of it before that time. It is quite understandable that a patient who recounts that sort of story to his doctor may be suspected of having had a stroke.

Whereas the sudden development of weakness or other symptoms reflecting troubles in the nervous system tends to suggest a stroke, a slow, gradual, progressive development of symptoms suggests the possibility of some progressive trouble in the nervous system, such as a slowly growing tumor. The doctor may have some difficulty in deciding which of these serious possibilities is most likely, especially in patients with no tremor. Even if there is tremor (not just any tremor but the *resting* tremor typical of Parkinson's disease), however, the doctor may want to be sure he is indeed dealing with Parkinson's disease and not a stroke or a brain tumor mimicking Parkinson's disease. He may order some neurological tests or refer the patient to a neurologist for a consultation.

The popular image of the specialist as an expert who can make the diagnosis of exotic diseases after briefly glancing at the patient

is a gross exaggeration. Of course, that does happen on occasion—
some conditions, though rare, are readily identified when first seen.
Parkinson's disease, when fully developed, is easily recognized.
The consultant's task is not merely to make the diagnosis or confirm
the referring doctor's impressions but to make sure that what seems
to be parkinsonism is not something else. There is no need for haste.
Parkinson's disease is not an acute illness nor is it life-threatening.
There is ample time to allow the consultant to consider the matter
as thoroughly as necessary.

The most important element in making a medical diagnosis is the
patient's own account of the symptoms. This account, called the
"history," is more important than all the tests modern laboratory
technology has made possible. It is even more important than the
physical examination itself. The consultant may ask numerous questions in order to gain an idea of the way in which the symptoms
developed. Some questions may seem silly or vague, and patients
sometimes answer facetiously or try to guess what is in the physician's mind and so give the answers they think he wants to hear.
Obviously, it is best to answer as directly and accurately as possible.
After all, the consultant can make a more accurate diagnosis when
he has reliable and correct information with which to work.

The neurological examination is a variety of the familiar physical
examination we undergo during an annual checkup or a pre-em-
ployment "physical." A complete neurological examination can be
a time-consuming affair. The routine "neurological" commonly done
by practicing neurologists may require 30 to 45 minutes or more,
depending on the circumstances. A great deal depends on simple
observation: By the time you have walked into the neurologist's
office and said "hello," he has already learned a number of important
things about you. During the formal examination conducted after
completing the "history," the neurologist examines the eyes, ears,
mouth, tongue, throat, and neck. He inspects and palpates the muscles in all four limbs and tests the strength of the muscles as well
as their tone. He uses the reflex hammer not only at the knee but
at other places as well: at the elbow, ankle, and maybe the jaw.
Every muscle has a reflex. The eye muscles are tested by studying

how the eyeballs move when you follow a moving object with the eyes. Your ability to perceive various sensations (such as pinprick, the touch of a twist of cotton, the vibration of a tuning fork, and others) is tested. The examination of sensory function is an important part of the neurological examination and can reveal some extraordinary things about "higher-level" function of the nervous system. Posture (sitting and standing), the character of your walk, the manner in which you get out of a chair, and the way in which you put on your clothes at the end of the examination are all observed. Finally, the neurologist usually administers some tests of mental function. These are generally simple items, such as a brief test of memory, abstract reasoning, and the ability to do simple calculations. He may ask you to repeat some numbers, spell some words, do some simple subtractions and multiplications, and perhaps interpret some old proverbs. These may seem silly and embarrassing but bear with it. The neurologist is not so much concerned with whether you answer correctly but the way in which you handle the task. It is also important for him to have some basic idea of the quality of your mental response to the ordinary problems we all have to handle every day. Most neurologists also ask for a sample of your handwriting.

The consultant is usually able to make a diagnosis or at least give a general outline of the problem and the measures that may be needed to pinpoint the diagnosis after completing the "history" and the neurological examination. He may say: "I believe you have Parkinson's disease, but I'd like to carry out certain tests to rule out some other possibilities." Perhaps your own doctor has already ordered these tests, and the consultant will want to review them before reaching a conclusion.

The neurological tests may include an x-ray of the head, an electroencephalogram, a radioactive brain scan, a computerized tomogram (the "CAT" or "CT" scan), as well as some blood tests. These tests do not require admission to hospital in ordinary circumstances and are usually done in the hospital outpatient department. The x-ray pictures of the head serve as a routine "screening" procedure. The chances of detecting a significant abnormality are small, but the test is harmless and a normal result is reassuring. The image cast on photographic film by the x-rays passing through the head can show only the bones or other structures containing calcium. The x-ray film does not reveal the brain itself, although it is sometimes possible for the radiologist interpreting the films to infer changes in the brain from indirect effects on the bone structure of the skull. Some brain tumors contain calcium and thereby reveal themselves on the x-ray. Also, certain structures in the brain normally contain enough calcium to be visible on an x-ray film. Calcium may also be deposited throughout the corpus striatum in some rare disorders of body calcium metabolism that can mimic Parkinson's disease.

The technique of computerized tomography (CT scan, for short) has proved to be a much more useful diagnostic test to evaluate patients with symptoms of brain dysfunction and has largely replaced the routine head x-ray films just described. The reason is that the CT scan actually shows the internal structure of the brain. We are mainly interested in detecting changes in the brain itself rather than in the skull, which is merely the box in which the brain is contained. The CT scan is a type of x-ray procedure, but instead of using photographic film to display the image, a series of images is constructed by a computer from a tremendous number of readings taken by radiation detectors. The patient's head is placed between an x-ray tube and a detector, both of which are mounted on a moving gantry in such a way that they can rotate about the head. The detector can make several hundred readings in precisely controlled positions. From the readings it is possible to calculate the intensity of the radiation at each of hundreds of points inside the head. A vast number of calculations must be done in order to determine the intensity at a sufficient number of points to produce an image. The calculations can be carried out within several minutes by a computer programmed for that purpose, and the computer then displays the image on a television screen. A series of images are normally obtained, and these are usually photographed on instant black and white film for study.

As a consulting neurologist, I have found the CT scan useful in studying patients I suspect of having Parkinson's disease or related conditions. It has the advantage of being able to detect not only tumors but also the scars of old strokes and changes in the structure of the brain which are characteristic of various disorders that can mimic Parkinson's disease. Thus, for example, it is helpful in distinguishing arteriosclerotic parkinsonism from Parkinson's disease.

The electroencephalogram is to the brain what the electrocardiogram is to the heart. Small electrodes temporarily attached to the scalp with glue detect electrical activities arising in the brain. The minute currents induced by brain activity in the scalp electrodes are magnified electronically (approximately 100,000 times) by an amplifier much like the amplifier in a high fidelity set. These activities are then recorded on moving paper so the patterns and rhythms can be analyzed. Abnormal patterns of activity occur in the presence of brain tumors, following strokes or other injuries to the brain, in certain drug and chemical intoxications, and in some persons with epileptic seizures. There are usually no characteristic changes in the electroencephalogram in Parkinson's disease. Thus a normal test serves as evidence against the possibility of tumor, stroke, or other brain disorders. The electroencephalogram, done here as a "screening" procedure, is harmless to the patient and may reveal valuable information. A normal reading, although not diagnostic, is reassuring.

The radioactive brain scan is a procedure in which a radioactive substance is given to the patient by injection. The substance then circulates throughout the body, including the brain. Radiation detectors placed around the head in a specially designed geometric pattern reveal a picture of the brain's circulation. The scan image can be caught on photographic film or displayed on a television screen. Most brain tumors absorb the radioactive material used in the test and thus are revealed in the scan image. It is also possible for this scan technique to give a fair idea of the adequacy of blood flow through the brain.

These several diagnostic procedures are commonly used to evaluate patients with symptoms indicating some disorder in the brain. All the tests are usually normal in cases of Parkinson's disease. The consultant considers the results of these tests, the history of the patient's symptoms, and the findings of the examination of the patient, and then arrives at the best possible diagnosis. Sometimes he asks for additional blood tests. Rarely, a case of parkinsonism with no tremor but only a general slowness in all bodily movement resembles a case of hypothyroidism. A few simple blood tests to measure the blood level of thyroid hormone are helpful in this circumstance. Usually he can say: "I believe you have Parkinson's disease" and can advise the patient on treatment. However, occasionally even the consultant with the benefit of all the tests described cannot make a diagnosis with certainty. He may wish to re-examine the patient in a month or two. This is not an unreasonable request. The consultant may need time to think about the case. Then too, the passage of time may allow the disease to reveal itself more clearly.

On several occasions over the years I have followed a given patient over a period of several months or even a year before I could make up my mind whether Parkinson's disease was really present. In one case, 2 years passed before I was certain of the diagnosis. The patient was a middle-aged woman who for several years had complained of pains in her legs while walking and of a sensation of burning in her legs and feet. She was thought to have some circulatory disturbance in her legs and was treated with various drugs to improve the circulation, to no avail. She was then noticed to have a mild tremor of the hands. I saw her in consultation. There was no rigidity, bradykinesia, or other signs of parkinsonism. The tremor was not of the "resting" type, and so I could not say with certainty that she had Parkinson's disease. I saw this patient again several times a year, and after 2 years I found some slight but definite rigidity in the arms and the tremor had become more typical of Parkinson's disease. It was then clear that the pains in her legs and the burning sensations were manifestations of Parkinson's disease and not of poor circulation. These symptoms disappeared on proper treatment of her parkinsonism.

Some physicians believe it best to reassure the patient with very early symptoms of Parkinson's disease that nothing is the matter. They fear that the very name "Parkinson's disease" will frighten and depress the patient, and so they try to reveal the diagnosis slowly or in stages. These physicians usually advise some responsible member of the family or the family doctor of the diagnosis. Sometimes the families join in this conspiracy of silence or insist on it themselves. I am often asked by concerned relatives not to tell the diagnosis to the patient. They slip me a note or call me in advance of a patient's appointment. "Mother doesn't know she has Parkinson's disease," they say, "Please don't tell her. We don't want her to know."

In rare circumstances there are good reasons for such silence, but in general I believe it is ill-advised. I have made a point of asking patients over the years how they felt about having the diagnosis of Parkinson's disease concealed from them. Invariably, they have been hurt and angered by the attempted secrecy. I say "attempted" because in most instances the deception failed. It did, however, often prevent the patient from getting answers to questions. Since the diagnosis could not be admitted, it could not be discussed. The patients have told me that they were not so much concerned with the name of the disease but that they wanted to know what to expect in the future, what treatment could be given, what the effects of treatment might be, and so on. They knew well enough that something was the matter, so protestations from the family and the doctor that nothing was the matter gave little comfort.

Once the diagnosis of Parkinson's disease is established and other possibilities excluded, the patient and doctor are ready to discuss the prognosis. Predicting the future is at best somewhat chancy, but some discussion about what the patient may expect, how his or her life is likely to be altered, what the treatment may be expected to accomplish, and so on is in order. Precisely what the diagnosis means to a given individual depends greatly, of course, on the person and the circumstances. Some patients, perhaps thinking of a relative or neighbor who may have had Parkinson's disease, may fear the worst and imagine that they will rapidly become severely invalid. This is, of course, an exaggerated view. In fact, the symptoms in most cases can be kept under good control for many years. Other patients may have a falsely rosy view. They may recall hearing about a new cure for Parkinson's disease or may have read a glowing newspaper account of a new drug treatment and are confident the doctor can make the whole thing go away with a few pills or injections. This is the other extreme.

Clearly it is important for the patient and the family to attain a realistic view of the nature of the disease and the general outlook. Patients should not hesitate to ask their doctor questions. To this end, both patient and family must allow the doctor to be as frank as possible.

Many patients spend much time and effort wondering about the origin of their disease. Often they ask if it could have been caused by some undue stress at work or at home, an accident, or some great personal grief. Questions along this line are quite understandable. They reflect the patient's attempt to grasp in some familiar or comprehensible form just what is happening. The fact that the cause of the disease is unknown makes such speculation inevitable. It is difficult for many to accept that in this age of incredible technical accomplishment we do not know the cause of this one disease or how to cure it. It is best to come to terms with this unfortunate reality in whatever way one can.

The disease *is* of unknown cause. It can be effectively treated but not cured. It progresses slowly, but successful treatment can control the symptoms for many years and allow the patient to lead an active and independent life. Hopefully, research may find improved means of treatment during the years ahead and make it possible to keep the symptoms reasonably in abeyance for the remainder of the patient's life.

CHAPTER 3

The Classic Triad

TREMOR

Of the three major symptoms of Parkinson's disease—tremor, rigidity, and bradykinesia—the most obvious and familiar is tremor. It is usually the symptom which first comes to the patient's attention and which most commonly brings the patient to a physician. The hand on one side is usually affected; sometimes one foot is involved. Typically the tremor occurs when the affected hand or foot is at rest. The shaking is regular and rhythmic, with a frequency of 5 to 6 beats per second. A simple, small to-and-fro motion of the arm or leg may be all that is obvious. More often, there is a complex movement, with slight turning of the forearm and a back-and-forth movement of the thumb and fingers reminiscent of a hand counting coins or of rolling a marble between the thumb and forefinger. For this reason, the tremor has been described as "pill-rolling" in quality.

The tremor disappears during sleep or when the patient is resting quietly. Thus it may be present only intermittently, and its presence reflects the patient's state of mind. Nervousness, being "under stress," or even the alertness induced by concentrating on a mental task regularly enhances the tremor. The patient may sit home reading the newspaper quietly and have no tremor at all until a visitor arrives. It is this aspect of the tremor which patients find socially embarrassing, and many avoid company for this reason.

Patients may feel the tremor even when it is too fine to be noticeable. It may be felt as a quivering or vibrating sensation. Tremor of the musculature of the abdomen is felt as something "quivering inside." Tremor of the diaphragm or of the chest muscles is sometimes felt as "palpitations," and the patient may fear erroneously that there is something the matter with the heart and so consult a physician for that complaint. Since the tremor can be detected by electrocardiography, it may obscure the electrical record of the heartbeat, making it difficult at times to evaluate the heart properly. The electrocardiogram may have to be repeated on another occasion.

Tremor may involve the tongue, lips, and jaw, but it rarely if ever causes shaking of the head; nor does tremor seem to affect the voice. Tremor may be confined to a very small part (for example, one finger). Some patients have told me their tremor began in the thumb or index finger!

A characteristic feature of tremor is its variability. It seems to come in bursts and then subside. The tremor of one part need not be synchronous with that in another. In fact, tremor may appear in a hand for a few minutes, then quiet down only to appear in the foot for awhile. Most patients are able to stop the tremor by an effort of the will. Many have learned various tricks to stop it. A slight movement or change of posture may arrest the tremor for awhile; eventually it reappears, after some minutes or sometimes longer.

Tremor in one hand while walking disappears if the patient remembers to swing the arm. It reappears when the patient forgets and allows the arm to hang idly at the side—as if tremor were a substitute activity. Holding something in the hand can also stop the tremor. One of my patients always carries a small package in one hand when out walking. He found that merely holding the small weight prevents the tremor, which he is anxious to conceal.

Many patients attempt to hide a trembling hand. They stuff the offending hand into a coat pocket, sit on the hand, or cover it with a newspaper or some object or even with the other, nontrembling hand.

Embarrassment at having a tremor is very common among Parkinson's disease patients. In contrast, however, persons with "essential tremor," which is usually more obvious and sometimes strikingly resembles the Parkinson tremor, do not seem to share this sense of embarrassment quite so often or so markedly. I have often pondered why one type of tremor was embarrassing and the other not. Patients have told me in response to my queries on this point that they are ashamed to appear ill to their friends or family. Others fear that colleagues at work or their boss might notice the tremor and draw unfavorable conclusions. Unfortunately, there may well be justification for the fear of letting "the boss" or clients or customers see the tremor. Doctors, lawyers, accountants, and other professionals with a Parkinson tremor often tell me their patients or clients seem to lose confidence in them after noticing the tremor. A clothing salesman was fired with the explanation that his tremor would make a poor impression on customers! On the other hand, many patients who were fortunate enough to work in family-owned businesses or who ran their own shops have continued their work successfully for years despite their tremor. There seems to be a need for better education of the public regarding Parkinson's disease.

In the very earliest phases of the disease, tremor sometimes occurs only at infrequent intervals, during periods of great nervous tension. For example, one patient first became aware of a tremor of the hand after an auto accident while trying to jot down the other driver's name, license number, and so on. The tremor subsided and did not reappear for several years! Understandably, the patient asked if the nervous strain of the accident might have caused Parkinson's disease in his case. It is not surprising that similar observations led 19th century medical writers to consider whether fright or "nervous exhaustion" might not indeed be a causative factor of Parkinson's disease. Now that we know much more about the organic basis of the symptoms of Parkinson's disease, we recognize that nervous tension may indeed increase the tremor or bring it out when it is otherwise not present, and it may even, in exceptional circumstances, reveal the tremor a few months or years before it might otherwise have been noted.

Tremor occurs in many conditions. One which is sometimes confused with Parkinson's disease is "benign essential tremor." Generally the tremor of this condition differs from that of Parkinson's disease in that it occurs not at rest but when the arms are held outstretched for a moment as when reaching for the handle of a teacup. It also differs in that essential tremor, unlike that of Parkinson's disease, often runs in families in a clearly hereditary pattern. However, the distinction based on the relationship of tremor to movement or position is not always so clear-cut. The major point of difference is that neither rigidity nor bradykinesia occurs in essential tremor. Thus a physician examining a patient who presents with the complaint of tremor does not try to reach a diagnosis from observation of the tremor alone. He looks for other signs—for the bradykinesia and rigidity—and does not make the diagnosis of Parkinson's disease until all three components of the classic triad are evident.

RIGIDITY

Patients often complain of a feeling of stiffness, which is perhaps their subjective appreciation of rigidity. Strictly speaking, rigidity is not a symptom the patient feels but an objective sign that can be appreciated only by another person physically examining the patient for evidence of resistance to passive motion. A physician takes the patient's arm and gently bends and straightens it a number of times while asking the patient to relax. The physician is looking for resistance to passive motion around the elbow joint. There may also be similar resistance to passive motion at other joints: the wrist, knee, ankle, spine, etc. A persistent resistance to such passive movement with a plastic quality is what we mean by the term *rigidity*. It has a very characteristic feel and cannot be voluntarily imitated by the patient. It differs from the type of resistance to passive motion encountered in spasticity. There is often a regular, jerky quality to the resistance as if there was a ratchet gear or cogged wheel in the joint being manipulated. Physicians know this as "cogwheel rigidity."

One can also see on looking at "rigid" muscles that they are constantly tensed in a state of sustained contraction when they should be soft and relaxed when not in use. The tightness and firmness of rigid muscles can be felt with the fingers.

The patient may be aware of the muscular rigidity not only as a sense of stiffness but as a tired, aching feeling, persistent soreness, a pain, or a cramp. Thus rigidity of the muscles of the head and neck is often experienced as a headache. Usually it is felt mainly in the back of the neck, shoulders, back of the head, and temples. Rigidity of the spinal muscles causes back pain (usually low back pain), which is aggravated by the tendency to stand leaning forward. Constantly leaning forward places the spinal muscles under a mechanical strain. Anyone who tries to stand leaning forward slightly in the posture common to many Parkinson patients soon experiences low back pain. Rigidity of the muscles of the calf and foot is manifested as painful cramps, not unlike the common "charley horse" provoked by athletic exercise.

Rigidity of the muscles of the chest and shoulder is sometimes felt as chest pain. When this occurs on the left side, the pain may be misinterpreted as the pain of heart disease known as "angina pectoris." I have known a number of patients who were unnecessarily frightened by such pain in the chest. One patient visited many heart specialists who, after numerous tests, could find nothing wrong with his heart. When he eventually developed some tremor and rigidity in the left hand, the diagnosis of Parkinson's disease could be made, and it became apparent that the chest pain was a symptom of Parkinson's disease. It disappeared after treatment with levodopa.

Aspirin and similar ordinary pain-relieving medications usually do not provide much help for the pain associated with sustained muscle contraction. Physical measures such as heat and massage are often helpful, at least temporarily; the back pain may be relieved by a hot bath, a back rub, or a heating pad applied to the muscles of the back. Massaging the muscles of the neck relieves headache, and kneading the calf muscle may relieve leg cramps. Proper treatment of the parkinsonism gives the best and most lasting relief. Improvement of the posture is also important in alleviating back pain. The pain often disappears immediately when the patient makes the effort to stand erect. A problem here is that the patient soon reverts to a stooped posture and again has back pain. Exercises to improve the posture are thus helpful but must be performed regularly to obtain good results.

BRADYKINESIA

Muscular rigidity slows movement. Some years ago many physicians believed that tremor and rigidity accounted for all the symptoms of Parkinson's disease. Rigidity may indeed impede movement. All movement requires the cooperation of opposing muscles—some relaxing while others contract and vice versa. The failure of an antagonist muscle to relax obviously limits a given movement. Consider a simple movement such as bending the arm (Fig. 3). The biceps muscle brings about the movement by contracting or shortening; it is the *agonist* in this case. The triceps muscle relaxes and allows itself to be stretched as the arm bends at the elbow, and it is the *antagonist* muscle here. To straighten the arm, the reverse occurs: the triceps contracts and biceps relaxes. Failure of the reciprocal action of these muscles (that is, failure of the triceps to relax on bending the arm, or failure of the biceps to relax on attempting to straighten the arm) is the essential feature of rigidity. It is the failure of reciprocal relaxation of antagonist muscles that the physician feels as a resistance to passive manipulation of the patient's limbs. The rigidity impedes not only passive movement but active movement willed by the patient as well. It seems readily understandable that rigidity has been blamed for the slowness of movement of parkinsonism (that is, for the bradykinesia).

The reality is more complicated. If patients are observed carefully, it can be seen that slowness of movement may occur in the limbs with the least rigidity, and that rapid movement can occur even with rigidity. Rare patients are observed who have bradykinesia but no rigidity at all. Thus the two major symptoms do not parallel each other. Physicians once debated this subject at some length. It was the experience with stereotactic brain surgery that finally convinced skeptics of the importance of bradykinesia. Many patients had excellent relief of tremor and rigidity, but in some cases relief of rigidity did not result in a corresponding reversal of bradykinesia.

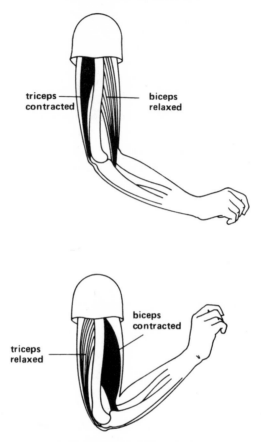

FIG. 3. Reciprocal action of agonist and antagonist muscles acting in opposing directions across a joint—in this case, the elbow joint.

Rigidity was abolished, but good, rapid movement was not necessarily restored.

I am sometimes surprised to see a patient who looks rigid but in whom I can find no signs of true rigidity (that is, of increased resistance to passive movement). This misleading appearance of rigidity is due to the complex phenomenon called bradykinesia or, more simply, akinesia (literally, absence of movement). The term refers to both slowness and poverty of movement. When bradykinesia is minimal, it is barely noticeable and may pass for normalcy.

Some persons are slower in movement than others; some are "poker-faced" quite normally, others are very expressive. Since the range of normalcy is broad, a mildly bradykinetic parkinsonian patient, especially if elderly, is apt to pass for normal. Persons close to the patient, however, may have noticed a change. A man who was formerly quick and vivacious who has now become slow and deliberate may still be within the range of normal to a casual observer, but those who know him well are aware of an appreciable change.

Perhaps one of the commonest manifestations of bradykinesia is the loss of automatic movements. These are movements we normally make without being conscious of them; they occur automatically. They include the associated movements of walking, eye blinking, swallowing of saliva, expressive movements of the face and hands, minor movements of postural adjustment and so on.

A normal person who is sitting is not actually perfectly still. The eyes blink spontaneously a number of times a minute. We are usually unaware of this occurrence or pay it little attention. The motor act occurs automatically without our consciously commanding it. Similarly, we swallow our saliva several times a minute. We shift our weight from one side to the other, cross our legs, maybe even do little fidgety movements such as tapping the floor with our foot or drumming on the arm of a chair with our fingers. We turn our head and eyes from side to side to survey the scene around us. We clear our throats, nervously cough, rub our necks, scratch here or there. All these movements are done without significant conscious participation. A striking feature of the severely bradykinetic Parkinson patient is that these spontaneous motor acts are done much less frequently than normal. There is thus a *poverty* of spontaneous movement.

The reduced frequency of eye blink gives the face a staring exprssion. The eye blink functions as a sort of windshield wiper, removing bits of dust settling on the surface of the eyes. With reduced blinking, the cleansing function is less effective and the eyes may become irritated. The eyelids become dry, reddened, and crusted, and the patient may experience a burning feeling in the eyes. Irrigating the eyes with artificial tears or a suitable eyewash several times a day usually alleviates this problem.

The diminished frequency of swallowing allows saliva to pool in the throat. When this is severe, saliva may spill forward in the mouth and pass through the lips, resulting in drooling. It was once thought that Parkinson patients produced abnormal amounts of saliva, but measurements have shown that this is not so. In fact, they produce normal amounts but simply do not swallow it at the normal rate. Treatment with anti-Parkinson drugs improves the rate of swallowing and also reduces the volume of saliva produced. The old "anticholinergic" drugs employed before levodopa was available dried up the saliva. Drooling was controlled but often at the expense of a feeling of dryness of the mouth.

Another class of automatic movements are those associated with walking. Normally, one swings the arms while walking, each arm in synchrony with the opposite leg. Also, when turning, one "leads" with the head. The head and eyes turn first, followed by the shoulders, and later the trunk and legs. The bradykinetic patient fails to swing the arms or swings them to a lesser extent and fails to lead with the head on turns. Instead, the body turns in one piece.

Bradykinesia is also apparent in more voluntary movements. Here it is seen as a hesitation in initiating an action, then a slowness in the movement, and finally rapid fatigue, which is especially evident in repetitive movements. These features may occur in many kinds of motor acts. For example, if walking is affected, there is a delay in starting to walk. The feet seem glued to the floor. Finally, after several false starts, the severely affected patient walks slowly with shuffling steps. The steps become progressively shorter and then walking suddenly stops. Bradykinesia may be demonstrated in an affected hand by asking the patient to tap the knee alternately with the palm of the hand and the back of the hand. After a few false starts, the patient taps satisfactorily if somewhat more slowly than with the other hand. Then the tapping becomes slower, and finally it stops as the patient seems unable to turn his hand over fully.

Common problems caused by bradykinesia include difficulty getting up from a chair, trouble getting out of a car, turning over in bed, donning a coat or jacket. The activity begins all right but slows down and falters just before it is successfully completed. It is as if

the energy required for the activity suddenly fails. Patients sometimes remark that they felt as if their batteries had run down. Other
patients feel the bradykinesia as an external force restraining their
movement. This is graphically shown in the self-portrait by an artist
patient shown in Fig. 4. The patient has drawn ropes shackling her
limbs to indicate her subjective experience of bradykinesia. Bradykinesia is also experienced as weakness or fatigue. It seems that the
actions rendered difficult by bradykinesia can nonetheless be accomplished by an effort of the will. This may seem fine to the
person observing the patient, and one is tempted to encourage the
patient by saying, "You see, you *can* do it all right." To the patient,
though, it seems that something which should be done easily and
without a thought requires effort and constant attention. One patient
complained to me that getting out of a deep, upholstered chair
required "a campaign of instruction to every muscle involved."

Another aspect of bradykinesia is a difficulty doing two things
simultaneously and in stopping one activity to start another. This
is perhaps just another aspect of the need to concentrate on an
ongoing activity to ensure its proper execution. Ordinary activities
such as dressing and eating therefore take longer than normal and
appear to be done in a deliberate manner.

Bradykinesia varies considerably from moment to moment and
in different circumstances. The patient can carry out an action or
movement on one occasion but not on another. The variation is
often quite striking in degree. The most striking examples are known
as *paradoxical kinesia*.

Every trace of parkinsonism seems to disappear for a brief period.
The phenomenon is especially striking in severely affected patients.
A chronic invalid who normally can barely walk with assistance
suddenly walks down the hall normally, or a very ill patient requiring
help to bathe and dress is found to have inexplicably gotten up early
and dressed entirely alone. Understandably, such variability in performance strains the credulity of the patient's family or attendants.
They are apt to refuse a later request for help in some minor task
and say: "You did it this morning all by yourself, why can't you

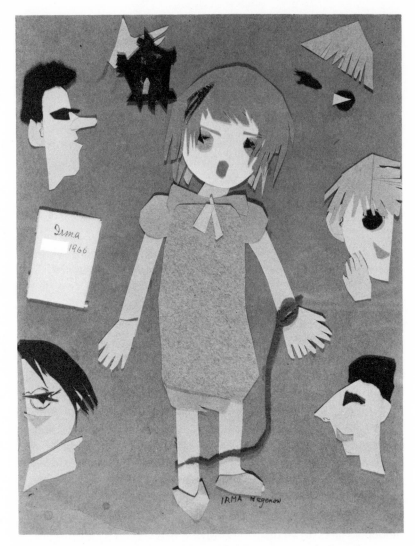

FIG. 4. Self-portrait of parkinsonism in collage by artist-patient.

do it now?" Alas, the patient cannot do it now and cannot explain why not. This is a common phenomenon in Parkinson's disease, but its mechanism is not known.

The phenomenon itself has been interpreted as evidence that the parts of the nervous system which control and coordinate all "motor" activity are intact, that they can function normally if properly activated. The basic problem, then, must be in some defective regulation of those parts of the brain. Here we are at the core of the problem of parkinsonism, for bradykinesia is surely the most important even though it is not the most obvious symptom. It is also the most difficult to understand.

Many thoughtful physicians have tried to analyze bradykinesia. One of the great neurologists of the first quarter of this century, Dr. S. A. Kinnier-Wilson, thought of the parkinsonian bradykinesia as a sort of "paralysis of the will." He came to this strangely metaphysical speculation because of the sense of effort and fatigue of which his patients complained. Such speculation, however, interesting though it might seem, does not help very much. What does "will" really mean? What connection is there between the material structure of the brain and a mental attitude or function such as "will"?

Other physicians saw patients' complaints that "everything becomes an effort" in another light. They argued that action was being blocked by some dysfunction in the brain. Far from the patients' lacking will power, they were in fact forced to rely on will power to overcome some central blocking or inhibiting effect. One eminent neurologist poetically observed that the patients were "condemned to voluntary movement." It has been noted that in general it is the automatic acts of daily life which are most affected by bradykinesia, and "learned" acts less so. Hence a severely bradykinetic patient may play the piano very well or execute a tap dance.

Leaving these interesting exceptions aside, however, every kind of activity may be affected by bradykinesia. It is hardly possible to describe all the specific manifestations of bradykinesia here. We can, however, take note of the basic elements of bradykinesia in whatever part of the body or type of activity is affected in a given patient at a given time.

CHAPTER 4

A Plethora of Symptoms

There are so many symptoms of Parkinson's disease it is difficult to mention them all in one volume. Many are uncommon or even rare, and few patients ever experience them. Some are fairly common but are more in the nature of nuisances than a serious cause of discomfort or disability. Understanding their mechanism and significance renders them innocuous, although, to be frank, symptoms that seem minimal to one patient may be severe and distressing to another.

Many symptoms are only special instances of tremor, rigidity, or bradykinesia. Some of these were discussed in the preceding chapter. We can usually understand the mechanism of these symptoms quite readily, and understanding often reduces them to the level of being a mere nuisance. Other symptoms are not so easily explained. We may simply have no real knowledge of their mechanism except that they are bona fide manifestations of Parkinson's disease.

ACHES AND PAINS

Parkinson's disease does not cause pain that requires a narcotic agent or powerful analgesic drug for relief. A variety of minor aches and pains do occur, however, and in extreme cases they can be quite distressing. Perhaps the most frequent symptom is an ache or soreness in an arm or leg which seems to be due to tremor and rigidity. The constant motion of tremor may represent a considerable amount of work done by the muscles of the affected limb, and it is

40

understandable that the symptoms of muscular fatigue are occasionally experienced. This may not be the only explanation, however; patients may experience this symptom when tremor and rigidity are barely noticeable but not at times when the tremor is more prominent. A sense of aching soreness may precede the first appearance of tremor by a year or more and then disappear.

A persistent nagging muscle ache may accompany pronounced muscle rigidity. This too may be explained by the considerable work the involved muscles do in sustaining a constant state of contraction. In neck muscles rigidity is experienced as headache, and in the foot or leg as a cramp. Usually foot cramps occur during the night or on first arising in the morning. Foot cramps while walking are someti.nes the initial symptom of parkinsonism. During the cramp the muscles of the foot and calf of the leg are in spasm and cause the toes to bend in a claw-like position. This can be quite uncomfortable, especially inside a tight shoe. Rarely, similar cramps affect the hand. Such a cramp provoked in the hand by tasks requiring fine control such as writing has been termed, aptly enough, "writer's cramp." There are, of course, many causes of writer's cramp, parkinsonism being only one among many and a rare one at that.

Aching low back pain is not uncommon in patients who tend to stand slightly stooped over. It is surprising how quickly the pain disappears when the patient stands truly erect or lies down; the pain may be worse in the sitting position because forward inclination of the back may be more marked in that position. Clearly, posture as well as muscle rigidity plays a role in this complaint. It is reminiscent of arthritis and is often erroneously ascribed to that disorder, but the usual remedies for arthritis—aspirin, salicylates, and simple analgesics—do not help, whereas they are quite useful to patients who really have symptoms referable to arthritis.

In addition to these various disagreeable sensations arising in muscles, some patients complain of a feeling of cold or, more often, warmth in some part of the body. It may be a hand, foot, the throat, or one side of the body, or it may seem to be internal, as in the stomach or rectum. I know a patient who for several years has experienced a feeling of coldness in his left hand. The feeling comes and goes irregularly; it may be absent weeks at a time and then appear once or twice a day. He wears a glove when the feeling appears. I have examined his hand at times when he was feeling the coldness. The hand felt cold to him, although its temperature felt completely normal to me. There was no discernible difference in skin temperature between the two hands! Another patient complained for several years of having cold feet at night. He put on wool socks before going to bed every night, even during the summer. The symptom eventually disappeared and has not recurred in many years.

A feeling of warmth is more common. Some patients experience a burning feeling in one hand or foot. An older woman who has had Parkinson's disease nearly 20 years complains to me frequently of a burning feeling in her throat and stomach. Extensive examinations have failed repeatedly to reveal any cause. She has had many x-ray studies of her esophagus and stomach. There is no ulcer or the slightest hint of inflammation. The stomach functions properly. There is, however, a connection between the symptom and her other symptoms. When for one reason or another her medications fail to take proper effect, her parkinsonism symptoms recur heralded by the burning feeling, which simulates a heartburn. Tremor, rigidity, and trouble walking soon follow. Adjustment of the medication invariably results in disappearance of the burning feeling and improvement of all the other symptoms.

These strange temperature sensations were described more than a hundred years ago as "thermal paresthesias." The medical word paresthesia means an abnormal sensation. The cause of these sensations is not known except that they are genuine albeit rare manifestations of Parkinson's disease. There is no specific treatment for this symptom; generally it responds to treatment of the parkinsonian state as a whole.

CHANGES IN POSTURE

Many patients with Parkinson's disease tend to stand in a mildly stooped posture. James Parkinson specifically mentioned this tendency in his introductory definition of *shaking palsy*. He described it as a "propensity to bend the trunk forwards" while standing and walking (Fig. 5). Not all patients develop this posture, and in many it is barely noticeable. Occasional patients also have a tendency to lean slightly to one side. It is especially noticeable in the sitting position.

Another common change in posture is a tendency to carry one arm bent at the elbow while standing or walking. If the patient makes an effort to swing the arm when walking, the posture disappears. It reappears as soon as the patient forgets to swing the arm.

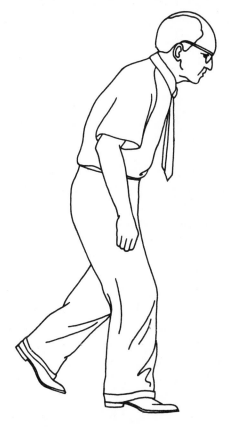

FIG. 5. Parkinson patient exhibiting typical "propensity to bend the trunk forwards" while walking, as described by James Parkinson.

A less common postural change is a tendency to hold the foot turned in slightly. This is usually most evident in the sitting position with the legs at rest. Sometimes it can be noticed when walking.

Characteristically, patients are not aware of these changes in posture. They are sometimes quite surprised when they see evidence of their posture in a mirror or in a reflection in a window. This is not true of all patients, however. Some are acutely aware of the changes in their posture, and it is these patients who are, of course, in a better position to do something to minimize these postural abnormalities with exercise and by sheer force of will.

PARKINSONIAN SPEECH

Many patients have no change in the character of their speech even after many years of Parkinson's disease, whereas in others the speech may be affected in a characteristic way. Rarely, it is the initial symptom. The first change is usually a tendency to speak softly. The patient may have difficulty being understood on the telephone. Strangely, patients are often unaware that their speech is soft and are perplexed that others have difficulty hearing them. A loss of the normal volume of speech may not be troublesome to some patients, whereas it is very important to others. It depends to some extent on the patient's life and work. A teacher, lawyer, actor, or someone who needs to speak or lecture notices the change in speech long before patients in other walks of life.

Some years ago I had a patient who was a college professor. His major problem was that his speech was not sufficiently loud to be heard in a classroom. When he lectured, the students could not hear him, although his diction was fine. Since he simply could not project his voice any more, he took a course of speech training exercises. This helped for a few years, but the students still complained that they could not hear his lectures. Finally, he obtained a throat microphone and a public address system. With electronic amplification of his voice, he was able to go on lecturing for many more years.

Another change in the character of speech is a tendency to talk in a steady, measured beat—in a careful, deliberate manner. Neurologists call this "monotone" speech. The "natural song" and cadence of speech seems to be lost.

Some patients speak not only softly and in a monotone but also rapidly. The words are crowded together without the usual pauses between phrases, and the syllables are run together. When these three features appear together, the resulting *soft, monotone, rapid* speech is so characteristic that the doctor should immediately think of Parkinson's disease.

Some patients, however, speak slowly instead of rapidly. Occasionally the voice becomes lower in tone (that is, hoarse), and occasionally higher in pitch. A rare phenomenon is a tendency to repeat a particular syllable in the middle of a word several times. It is similar to stammering but yet is different in character. The medical term for this is *palilalia*.

All of these changes in speech are improved by effective drug therapy. They were not helped by the once-practiced surgical operation for Parkinson's disease; in fact, the operation often made speech worse.

The softness of parkinsonian speech is due to a diminished movement of the chest. Normally, the chest acts as a bellows, forcing air through the larynx (the voice box) to produce the sound of speech, which is then modulated by the throat, mouth, tongue, and lips to form words (that is, speech). Both rigidity of the chest muscles and bradykinesia affecting the whole action account for the diminished volume of speech. The rapid pace of monotone speech in parkinsonism is more difficult to explain, but essentially the same thing occurs in such other activities as walking, writing, and actions requiring repetitive movements. The tendency to diminished use of facial expressive movements and hand gestures while talking may further hinder the patient's ability to communicate.

SWALLOWING

Akin to the problems of speech are changes in swallowing. The two, however, do not necessarily accompany one another. Swallowing is also a very complex act, although it is performed automatically. In Parkinson's disease, the complex sequential pattern of contraction and relaxation of the throat muscles necessary to propel food particles to the rear of the throat and into the esophagus may be slowed. The rate of swallowing is decreased. Consequently, eating may become slower and assume a deliberate quality. The patient must wait until the last morsel of food goes down before attempting to swallow the next. Food seems to be held up at the top of the throat. Liquids and solids are equally difficult to swallow; soft foods seem to go down more readily. Attempts to hurry only make matters worse. Usually it is necessary only to be patient and to eat slowly but steadily.

Slowing of the normal automatic act of swallowing one's saliva results in a pooling of saliva in the mouth and throat. When a large amount is allowed to accumulate, it may spill forward between the lips. The patient is then said to drool. Many patients feel that an excessive amount of saliva is flowing or being produced. However, careful measurements of salivary flow have shown that, in fact, these individuals form no more saliva than anyone else. Drooling occurs only because the patient fails to swallow at the normal rate. The drug treatment of parkinsonism usually results in both improved swallowing and a reduced production of saliva.

TROUBLE WALKING

Rather characteristic changes in the manner of walking occur in many cases of parkinsonism. The gait is generally less lively, the step shorter, the foot is not raised to the usual height, and the automatic swing of the arm in time with the opposite leg is diminished or lost. Turns are negotiated slowly, sometimes with hesitation and with the body moving in one piece, whereas normally the head turns first to be followed by the trunk and then the legs. When walking is more markedly involved, the toe may not be raised off the floor, and the patient consequently shuffles with one or both feet.

When walking is more severely impaired, several strange things occur. One may be called "freezing." The patient may be walking along very nicely when suddenly one foot seems to stick to the floor, firmly glued. After a few seconds it is suddenly loose again. This annoying phenomenon may occur very rarely or frequently. A curious feature is that freezing tends to occur especially in doorways, while crossing the street, and on turns. When severe, it may precipitate a fall.

When the freezing phenomenon is prominent, the patient may have difficulty initiating the act of walking when first arising from a chair or getting out of bed. A number of very short steps, of an inch or so, are all that can be accomplished, and then suddenly the patient steps out with a normal step and walks normally across the room. The neurologist describes this pattern of rapid, short, shuffling mini-steps as *festination*.

When long runs of festination appear, the patient may lean forward further and further as the steps become progressively faster and shorter until, after a dozen steps or so, the patient falls forward unless caught by someone or saved by some suitable obstacle. Some patients are able to use a cane effectively to stop the forward rush. The entire phenomenon is known as *propulsion*. When it occurs with backward stepping, it is called *retropulsion*. For example, the patient may make a few involuntary backward steps when backing out of a closet after hanging up a coat or when turning around a corner. For patients prone to retropulsion, wearing shoes with high heels may diminish or prevent the backward stepping.

The reasons for these disturbances of walking are not fully understood. Part of the problem appears to be an impairment of equilibrium. Walking has been described as a sort of controlled falling forward, each step being a response to an impending fall. A common feature of patients having these problems is a diminished response to an impending fall. The normal responses to an impending fall are made too late, too slowly, and with movements too small. The normal responses—stepping, flinging the arms, and adjusting the position of the head and trunk—are normally done very rapidly and instinctively or automatically. I often test patients in the office for their response to a sudden gentle shove forward or backward. When suddenly pushed backward, the normal subject simply steps back, flings the arms forward, and bends the head and trunk forward. The parkinsonian patient with walking problems and poor equilibrium, on the other hand, fails to do these things and instead leans backward without stepping. If balance is especially poor, retropulsion may result (Fig. 6), or propulsion if the patient is pushed forward.

Usually these walking disturbances respond fairly well to proper drug treatment. If necessary, physical therapy with emphasis on gait

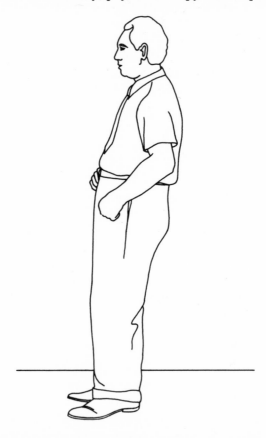

FIG. 6. Unaware that he is leaning backward, this patient thinks he is standing erect. He is about to step backward involuntarily in the phenomenon of retropulsion.

training exercises may help. Shoes with rubber soles that do not slide easily on the floor may greatly increase the patient's difficulties.

CHANGES IN BOWEL HABITS

Slowness of movement seems to affect the bowels as well as the limbs and all bodily movements generally in parkinsonism. Constipation is a common and recurrent problem for many patients. Several factors may contribute to this. Many patients eat poorly, neglecting roughage and drinking little water. As a result, their stools become small, rough, and hard. This may make bowel movements painful and exacerbate any hemorrhoids that might be present. Constipation is usually only a nuisance, but careful attention to maintaining proper bowel habits fully rewards the little effort required.

SLUGGISH BLADDERS

Less frequently, there may be some sluggishness of the bladder musculature so that urination may also be slowed. There may be difficulty in properly emptying the urinary bladder, and the patient may thus have to void again after a short time. Sometimes the patient allows the bladder to overfill, and then suddenly there is an overwhelming urgency to void right away. This is especially annoying at night, for it may necessitate getting up several times. Serious disturbance of bladder function is rare in Parkinson's disease. Should it occur, some other problem should be suspected, such as enlargement of the prostate gland in males or infection of the bladder or a "dropped" bladder in females.

SEXUAL DYSFUNCTION

Human sexual function is complex and intertwined with every aspect of life. It is a many-splendored thing, but it is also very intimate and personal; difficult to discuss with a stranger, even a physician. Perhaps this is why few patients complain of sexual dysfunction and why little is known of sexual problems in parkinsonism. Unfortunately, there have been few systematic studies of the problem.

The nervous system is involved in sexual activity at every level, from the highest to the lowest. Consequently, the nervous control of sexual function is susceptible to disruption at many points. At the highest level, psychological factors profoundly affect sexual behavior. For example, depression, anxiety, and frustration provoked by the very fact of being ill may sharply curtail libido. This is a common reason for sexual difficulties in many chronic disorders. Libido may be selectively impaired in parkinsonism by the disease process itself. Dopamine nerve cell systems in the brain seem to play some role in regulating libido. Patients have been described who have parkinsonism, loss of the sense of smell, and decreased libido. All three were improved by L-DOPA treatment. Although this combination of symptoms has not been systematically studied in Parkinson patients, clinical experience suggests that it does occur in a small but significant number. The improvement of libido on L-DOPA treatment has been well-documented, and is discussed in the chapter on L-DOPA. It may be partial, satisfactory, or perhaps sometimes excessive. Spouses have occasionally complained of exaggerated libido in patients when L-DOPA treatment is first undertaken.

Rarely, the nervous system is affected at a lower level, and the nerves directly controlling the sexual organs may be involved. The result is difficulty in maintaining a penile erection in the male and delayed ejaculation. Comparable problems presumably may arise in female patients, but so far no evidence on the subject is available. These difficulties are often accompanied by other manifestations of disturbance in the nerves controlling vegetative functions; notably, impaired control of blood pressure, the urinary bladder and the bowel, and loss of sweating in the legs. This complex of symptoms develops mainly in some of the atypical forms of parkinsonism that I have called "parkinsonism plus" and is especially found in the Shy-Drager syndrome. Indeed, in that condition, impotence without loss of libido may be the initial symptom. I can recall several patients who had experienced this phenomenon for 1 or 2 years before any sign of parkinsonism was evident. They had sought help at clinics specializing in the treatment of sexual dysfunction, to no avail. Unfortunately, this type of difficulty is not helped by L-DOPA or other therapies.

Limitations of bodily movement imposed by rigidity and brady-kinesia may cause problems simply by complicating the mechanical aspects of love-making. For example, slowness in turning over in bed may make it difficult for an affected male partner to assume a good position for foreplay or coitus. Rigidity and bradykinesia may hinder the pelvic movement necessary for coitus. Some accommodation to these difficulties can be made with some forethought and the assistance of an understanding spouse, but they nevertheless deprive the patient and his spouse of the natural spontaneity of normal love. Improvement of rigidity and bradykinesia on L-DOPA treatment restore normal sexual activity, chiefly by removing these mechanical impediments.

Many commonly used drugs, notably tranquilizers, antidepressants, muscle relaxers, and simple sedative and sleep medications may impair sexual function. The anticholinergic anti-Parkinson drugs may also do this to some extent, at least in some patients. Usually these drug effects result in delayed ejaculation and impairment of penile erection. Thus, if a sudden change in sexual function has occurred, it is well to consider whether it followed a change in drug treatment.

Many patients are afraid to discuss their sexual problems with their physicians (and vice versa). They tend to accept them as inevitable accompaniments of their condition, or as a natural result of aging. But such may not be the case. Sexual dysfunction may be secondary to drug therapy, or may result from an unrelated problem. Awareness of a problem may alert the physician to avoid certain drugs in planning treatment. I would urge patients and their spouses to overcome their natural reticence, and freely discuss sexual dysfunctions with their doctors.

LOW BLOOD PRESSURE

In most patients blood pressure is quite normal. Indeed, in my experience hypertension occurs less frequently among Parkinson patients than among other persons of the same age. However, a small number of patients may have low blood pressure. The sympathetic nerves which regulate the heart and blood vessels and thus determine the blood pressure are known to be affected in Parkinson's disease. If the involvement is sufficiently severe, low blood pressure may result, especially when the patient stands up. That is, the pressure may be normal when the patient is in the sitting position but drops to a low level on standing. For that reason it is referred to as *postural* hypotension.

It is very rare for Parkinson patients to be aware of this low blood pressure, and it is not often recognized because blood pressure is usually measured in the sitting position only. However, if the blood pressure is sufficiently low, symptoms of weakness, faintness, dizziness, light-headedness, etc. may be experienced on standing or walking, especially when first arising after sitting or lying for a time. The tendency to postural hypotension is exaggerated by drug treatment, especially with levodopa. It is usually easily controlled by various measures, which are discussed in the chapter on levodopa.

SWELLING OF THE FEET

Swelling of the feet sometimes occurs, usually appearing first and to a more marked degree on the side of the body where the first symptoms of parkinsonism appeared many years earlier. Usually this occurs only in patients with a significant amount of bradykinesia. It seems to be due to diminished movement of the affected leg. The circulatory system relies on the effect of movement of the legs and contractions of the leg muscles to propel the blood in the veins upward toward the heart. If there is little motion, as in the patient who sits still all day, the veins in the legs become congested; some fluid then leaks out and accumulates in the tissues, chiefly in the feet and ankles.

This fluid accumulation is called *edema*. It tends to diminish overnight and to increase during the day. If one presses down firmly on the skin of the ankle with the tip of a finger, a small depression can be produced which persists for some time. Physicians often search for this sign of edema when examining patients whose ankles seem swollen.

The swelling itself is usually mild in Parkinson patients and has no sinister significance. Sometimes patients think their legs are heavy and ascribe their difficulty in walking to the swelling. Of course, their swollen feet have nothing to do with their problems in walking. Occasionally the swelling makes it difficult to put on tight shoes, but otherwise the problem is chiefly a matter of appearance, that is, "cosmetic."

The edema usually subsides after proper treatment of the parkinsonism and as the patient becomes more mobile and moves the legs more vigorously. Sometimes additional measures are employed, such as use of a diuretic drug.

SEBORRHEA

Excessive discharge of the oily secretion of the sebaceous glands of the skin commonly occurs in Parkinson's disease. The skin of the forehead, the face at the sides of the nose, and the scalp are particularly affected. The forehead appears oily or greasy all the time but more so in warm weather. The oily discharge may be irritating to the skin and cause redness, itching, and scaling. On the scalp the scaling is recognized as *dandruff*. When the irritation is sufficiently annoying, it may be termed *seborrheic dermatitis*. This is a common skin disorder that occurs in many people who do not have Parkinson's disease or any other disorder of the nervous system. Dandruff alone is even more common. The various treatments (chiefly detergents and soothing lotions) commonly used for dandruff and seborrheic dermatitis may be used as effectively in Parkinson patients as in others.

EXCESSIVE SWEATING

Excessive sweating is another common manifestation of Parkinson's disease. It may affect one side of the body or even just one area, but it is usually generalized. The excessive sweating tends to occur in irregular bursts. It seems that the sweat glands are somehow poorly controlled and may respond to normal stimuli in an exaggerated manner. The tendency to excessive sweating is usually greatly reduced by treatment of parkinsonism. The mechanism is not understood.

CONJUNCTIVITIS

The decreased frequency of eye blink may result in the annoying symptom of burning or itching of the eyes. The reason is that the normal "windshield wiper" function of the eyelids is not being carried out with the normal frequency. Thus dust particles, grit, smoke, and other irritants which are normally swept away with a blink are allowed to remain for an unduly long time. Consequently, the white of the eyes and the eyelids may become irritated. The eyes appear "bloodshot," and crusts form on the edges of the lids. Irrigating the eyes with artificial tear solutions usually relieves these symptoms quite readily.

HANDWRITING IN PARKINSONISM

Characteristic changes in handwriting that occur in Parkinson's disease may be of diagnostic value to the physician and a nuisance to the patient. The handwriting tends to get smaller. The letters are well formed but get progressively smaller as the patient continues to write; at the end, the letters may be so small as to be difficult to read. However, if one looks at the writing with a magnifying glass, the letters still seem well formed. This pattern may not be evident when writing only a few words or a signature, but if samples of the patient's signature several years back are examined, a change is often evident. The tendency to write small is called *micrographia*.

In addition, if one looks closely, tremor may be evident in the writing in the form of very small squiggles in each letter (Fig. 7).

Effective drug treatment of parkinsonism produces marked changes in handwriting. It may become normal again, or it may be over-corrected so that now the patient writes in an unusually bold, large hand with extravagant flourishes. This is characteristic of the hand-writing of patients with chorea and seems to parallel the appearance of drug-induced chorea, a subject discussed in the chapter on levo-dopa treatment.

VISUAL PROBLEMS

Occasionally patients with longstanding Parkinson's disease complain of difficulty reading. They consult an ophthalmologist or an optometrist but are told their eyes are normal. They may need a new set of reading glasses, but aside from this, no ocular abnormality is found. Tests of visual acuity are normal. Sometimes patients are advised that the medication given to treat their parkinsonism may be the cause of their visual problem. This is, however, usually not the case. The oculists are simply unable to explain the patient's complaint.

One reason for difficulty reading is that the eyes do not move properly to scan a line of print. The eyes move in an irregular, jerky manner—slowing here, jumping ahead there—so the patient has to work hard to make out the sequence of letters and words. Then, having reached the end of the printed line, the patient has difficulty moving the eyes back to the left and down one line to find the beginning of the next line. Reading thus becomes a laborious task, and the patient soon tires of it. The problem is not in the eyesight itself. The optical properties of the eye have not changed. The problem is impaired coordination of the muscles which move the

This is a sample of my beautiful handwriting

FIG. 7. Sample of handwriting showing micrographia and, if one looks carefully with a magnifying glass, evidence of tremor. Look especially at the "f" in beautiful.

eyeballs from side to side and up and down. That this is indeed the problem can usually be ascertained with a little thought and careful analysis. There seems to be an analogy between the disturbances in walking and those in eye movement in parkinsonism. The eyes festinate, freeze, and travel slowly across the printed page while reading.

A rare phenomenon, *ocular lateropulsion*, may occur in which the gaze tends to drift involuntarily to one side so the patient has difficulty directing his vision to the point he would like to see. This seems analogous to the disturbance in equilibrium and walking called *lateropulsion* in which the patient tends to veer to one side.

These disturbances in the coordination of the muscles which move the eyeballs are usually greatly benefited by levodopa therapy. However, they may not always be completely alleviated. Even so, marked impairment of eye movement is distinctly unusual in Parkinson's disease and, if unresponsive to treatment, suggests that a diagnostic re-evaluation is in order. If there is obvious impairment of eye movement, the diagnosis may need revision or else some other eye problem may have developed.

A very occasional patient with Parkinson's disease may experience double vision. That is, the patient sees two separate images of the world about him, one overlapping the other but separate, somewhat like the split image in a camera range-finder when the lens is out of focus. This is due to the fact that both eyes are not looking at precisely the same point. This ocular phenomenon was common in the postencephalitic form of parkinsonism but may also occur, although rarely, in Parkinson's disease and other forms of parkinsonism. The problem is probably in the nerve cells which control the muscles moving the eyeballs. A curious feature is that the double vision tends to fluctuate. It may be present on some occasions, absent on others, and may vary during the day from minimal to marked. Spectacles with special prisms may correct the double vision. However, due to the variability of the phenomenon, some patients are helped by prisms but others are not. Usually, in time, the patient becomes tolerant of the double vision. The brain learns to ignore one of the images, and double vision is no longer experienced, even though it can be demonstrated by appropriate testing of the eyes.

There seems also to be a more subtle problem with vision in some patients that may be described as an impairment of visual perception. That is, there is some problem in the interpretation of the image cast on the retina by the lens system of the eye. The nature and significance of this dysfunction is not understood and is the subject of current research. It was recently discovered that the retina has a special group of nerve cells which contain dopamine. The possibility arises that the retinal cells may be depleted of dopamine in Parkinson's disease. Whether such a depletion does in fact occur is not yet known, but it could explain some of the more subtle disturbances of vision that occur.

If one looks at a pattern of alternating light and dark bars, or at a flashing light, changes occur in the electrical activity of the brain that can be detected by electrodes placed on the back of the head over the part of the brain concerned with vision. These may be seen on the ordinary electroencephalogram (EEG), but computer analysis of the EEG is needed to sort out the visual effect from other electrical activities. The result is a characteristic pattern of activity called the *visual evoked potential* (VEP). The VEP is frequently abnormal in patients with Parkinson's disease. It is delayed and disorganized. The significance of this finding is uncertain, but it might be caused by depletion of retinal dopamine. It is interesting that the VEP returns toward normal after treatment with levodopa. Although many patients have an abnormal VEP, very few are aware of any impairment of vision; and they carry out ordinary activities of daily living without any evidence of defective vision or disturbance of visual perception.

CHAPTER 5

Principles of Treatment

*The desire to take medicine is perhaps
the greatest feature which
distinguishes man from animals.*

SIR WILLIAM OSLER

Over the long run, the patients who are the most successful in dealing with Parkinson's disease are those who enjoy a good working relationship with their physicians and families. The treatment of parkinsonism is necessarily more than the relief of specific symptoms. It is a cooperative undertaking, a joint enterprise of the patient, family, and doctor. Working together over the years, they seek to achieve not only the most satisfactory control of troublesome symptoms but also to make living with the disease as effective and successful as possible. Needless to say, the support and love of a concerned spouse, and of the family as a whole, make a great difference. Generally it is best to continue with one physician, preferably the family doctor or an internist who can assume overall responsibility for medical care, and to rely on specialist consultants only when the primary physician needs their help for diagnosis, for specific advice regarding treatment, and for special problems that may arise from time to time. Continuity of medical care with regular visits and periodic checkup examinations is of great importance in a chronic disorder such as Parkinson's disease. It is a deplorable waste of time for patients to hop about from one doctor to another looking for a better or a new treatment without giving each new doctor sufficient time to become acquainted with and to learn the

58

patient's individual reactions to the various treatments available. There are no secret treatments known only to one doctor or available only at a certain clinic or hospital.

There is no curative treatment for Parkinson's disease at the time I am writing this. Nor, to be realistic, is there any immediate prospect of a cure being found. Other forms of parkinsonism (such as postencephalitic or arteriosclerotic parkinsonism) cannot be cured. Of course, parkinsonism induced by tranquilizing drugs subsides when the patient stops taking the drug in question or even when the dose is reduced. In the rare instance of parkinsonism caused by a glandular disturbance, correcting the disturbance results in gradual disappearance of the parkinsonism. The cause of most forms of parkinsonism is unknown, and so treatment is symptomatic. That is, treatment alleviates the symptoms without attacking the disease process itself. However, the symptoms can be so well controlled that progression of the underlying disease may be effectively masked for many years. Patients often forget what having parkinsonism is like. Unfortunately, if they discontinue treatment, the symptoms recur. Thus treatment must be continued indefinitely—essentially for the remainder of the patient's life or until someone discovers a cure.

Treatment rests primarily on the use of various drugs, often two or more in combination. Physical therapy or informal exercise is often helpful and sometimes necessary. There is no specific dietary or vitamin therapy, although attention to one's general health and thus a proper diet is as beneficial to parkinsonian patients as to anyone else. Brain surgery to relieve tremor and rigidity was largely abandoned after the introduction of levodopa nearly a decade ago, although it is still useful in certain cases. An important element of treatment is the interpretation of symptoms, as well as the advice and reassurance that an understanding and knowledgeable doctor can provide. It is essential to adjust one's life to the reality of the disease. All these things are important, but in the final analysis the cornerstone of effective treatment is the proper use of various drugs.

I believe it is important that patients know something about their medication. They should understand why they are taking it and what results may be expected. They should be aware of the major side effects and how we can deal with them. With such knowledge, patients can often better cooperate with their doctor and so treatment can be more effective. However, treatment should be left to the physician. Self-treatment often leads to insuperable difficulties. Even patients who are themselves physicians should leave the treatment to another. An old aphorism has it that the doctor who treats himself has a fool for a patient and an incompetent for his physician. The wisdom of this familiar saying applies to all patients. Even if you do know something about the disease and its treatment, you cannot do a good job treating yourself. It is too difficult to judge objectively one's own responses to treatment and to observe accurately one's own symptoms.

In fundamental terms, the drugs currently available for the treatment of parkinsonism act either by replenishing brain dopamine, mimicking the action of dopamine, or by modifying the function of the brain in such a way as to compensate in some degree for the deficiency of brain dopamine. Dopamine is only one of many chemical messengers in the brain. Another messenger substance bears the chemical name acetylcholine. It is a very important substance. Indeed, there is much more acetylcholine in the brain than dopamine. It appears to be the chemical messenger for many nerve cell systems throughout the brain and is present in large amounts in the corpus striatum. Unlike dopamine, acetylcholine is not deficient in parkinsonism. On the contrary, there appears to be a reciprocal seesaw relationship between these two messengers and their respective nerve cell systems. It is believed that dopamine acts to restrain the acetylcholine nerve cells, and that in parkinsonism the acetylcholine nerve cells are released from this restraining influence. Their unrestrained and consequently improperly regulated activity contributes in some manner to the various symptoms. Drugs that block or inhibit the action of acetylcholine tend to ameliorate the symptoms, whereas drugs that act by enhancing or imitating the action of acetylcholine cause an increase of parkinsonian symptoms. The opposite occurs in the case of dopamine. Drugs which block the function of the dopamine nerve cells make parkinsonism worse or even produce the disorder, whereas drugs which enhance these nerve cells relieve the symptoms.

The drugs useful in the treatment of parkinsonism can be understood in terms of the seesaw reciprocal relationship of dopamine and acetylcholine. On the one hand are the drugs which block the action of acetylcholine. These are the *anticholinergic drugs*. On the other hand are the drugs which enhance or imitate the action of dopamine; we will call these *dopaminergic drugs*. A very large number of drugs can block acetylcholine, and a few of these are recognized as anti-Parkinson drugs. Their overall efficacy is limited. On average, they can reduce the intensity of the symptoms of Parkinson's disease approximately 20 to 25%. Their effect in postencephalitic parkinsonism is much greater, and they can completely abolish drug-induced parkinsonism. Several types of drugs can enhance the function of dopamine nerve cell systems. Perhaps one of the most familiar is amphetamine. However, amphetamine and its numerous cousins have very little effect in Parkinson's disease. They were useful years ago in combating the drowsiness and tendency to excessive sleep that was a frequent symptom of postencephalitic parkinsonism; they have no effect on drug-induced parkinsonism. Since amphetamines work indirectly by causing dopamine nerve cells to release dopamine, they might reasonably be expected to be ineffective when there is a deficiency of dopamine, and thus the poor effect of the amphetamines in parkinsonism need not be surprising. The most effective way of improving the function of the "sick" dopamine nerve cells is to replenish the depleted stores of dopamine. This is most easily accomplished by feeding patients the precursor substance L-DOPA, which is converted in the brain to dopamine. Drugs that mimic the action of dopamine are also useful in treating parkinsonism. They offer the theoretical advantage of not having to be converted in the brain to the active substance, but of acting directly on the dopamine receptors in the corpus striatum, in effect imitating or substituting for dopamine. They are called dopamine receptor agonists, they are less effective than L-DOPA, but more effective than the anticholinergics.

One drug widely used in treating parkinsonism, amantadine (Symmetrel) is difficult to classify because we are not sure just how it works. It does not seem to have direct acetylcholine-blocking properties and is thought by some researchers to act on the dopaminergic system. Probably it possesses indirect anticholinergic properties.

L-DOPA is the most effective agent available for the treatment of Parkinson's disease and most types of parkinsonism, with the exception that it does not reverse parkinsonism induced by the major tranquilizing drugs. Nevertheless, many neurologists prefer to treat early or mild cases of Parkinson's disease with one of the anticholinergic drugs or with amantadine, and reserve L-DOPA for more severe cases or for use at a later date when amantadine and the anticholinergics prove insufficient. Some fear that L-DOPA may accelerate the progression of the disease. The evidence presented in support of that view seems less persuasive to me than the contrary evidence presented by Dr. Charles Markham of the University at Los Angeles, based on long-term follow-up studies. It is difficult to make hard and fast rules about which course to follow that would be applicable to all cases. Both approaches are reasonable. The treating doctor must evaluate each case in the light of his or her personal experience.

SIDE EFFECTS

Whichever drugs or combination of drugs is employed, certain general patterns of response may be expected. Much depends on the precise dosage and timing of the drugs taken. With proper care and diligence on the part of both patient and doctor, very good results can be achieved in most cases. The relief of symptoms can be striking. Usually, however, some side effects may have to be accepted in exchange for the benefits. Naturally, some patients are more sensitive to the drugs than others. Some side effects are only mildly annoying whereas others can be quite distressing. Generally, the higher the dose, the greater are both the benefits and the side effects. The goal of treatment is to find the best possible compromise between the desired effects—that is, relief of parkinsonism—and the undesired or side effects.

We should distinguish side effects from adverse effects. *Side effects* are normal effects of a drug proportional to the dosage. Individuals vary considerably in responsiveness, and thus a given effect may occur at a low dose in some persons and at a high dose in another. In any single person, however, effects become greater as the dose increases. Some effects are desirable but only up to a point. After that, they are undesired, or side effects. For example, the reduction in salivary flow by anticholinergic drugs may be a desirable effect in a patient with excessive flow of saliva but at a higher dose or in another patient annoying dryness of the mouth may occur. This is then a side effect. By lowering the dose, the effect can be reduced to a desirable effect. In the same sense, we consider drunkenness a side effect of whiskey. One glass may produce a pleasant state of mind but a "higher dose" produces the "side effect" of intoxication.

Side effects can be serious, even life-threatening, with whiskey as well as with the various anti-Parkinson drugs. Thus careful adjustments of dosage is necessary to obtain the balance between desired and undesired effects best suited to each patient. To strike the right balance is not always an easy task. It cannot be done by the patient. It must be done by another person who can see the patient objectively, preferably a person who knows something about the chemistry of the drug, its toxicity, its interaction with other drugs, and how to manage side effects. In short, the regulation as well as the prescribing of drugs should be left to the physician. In my experience, the patients who derive the best results from drug treatment are generally those who follow their prescribed regimen consistently and precisely.

Adverse effects are undesirable reactions that occur only in some patients. Usually they are unrelated to dosage and are uncommon. They can be allergic reactions such as may occur with any drug or food; for example, the patient may develop an itchy red rash on the arms. Some adverse reactions are more serious, even life-threatening. When an adverse reaction occurs, the drug must be stopped.

After the reaction subsides, treatment may be resumed with another drug, preferably one that is chemically unrelated.

A third type of undesired effect is sometimes caused by the interference of one drug in the action or metabolism of another drug. Some examples of drug interaction are given later.

RESPONSE OF SYMPTOMS

The symptoms of Parkinson's disease are not all equally responsive to drug treatment. Some symptoms respond quite readily, others less so, and some not at all. In fact, some symptoms may be exacerbated. For example, the tendency to constipation common in Parkinson patients is increased by most of the anti-Parkinson drugs.

Patients often ask for a drug to control one symptom and another to ease another symptom, but the drugs do not work that way. It just is not possible to treat parkinsonism symptom by symptom. In general, the anti-Parkinson drugs act on the parkinsonian state as a whole, and they do not differ in their relative specificity for one or another symptom. It was once thought that some drugs were better for rigidity and others for tremor or akinesia. This line of thinking is reflected in the trade names of some drugs; for example, Akineton implies an action on akinesia, and Tremin suggests a special effect on tremor. Treatment based on such concepts led to complicated regimens with three, four, or even five drugs being given at the same time. Fortunately, these views have been largely abandoned; I say fortunately because side effects are more frequent with multiple drug regimens, and it is generally easier to adjust the dosage of one drug than of several. If excessive side effects or adverse effects develop, it may be difficult to judge which of several drugs is responsible and which to stop or reduce. In short, it is better to use one drug well than three not so well. It also is good practice as well as common sense to use as few drugs as possible in the lowest doses that give a satisfactory result.

Generally, rigidity is the most responsive symptom of the "classic triad" to drug treatment. With levodopa therapy it is usually completely abolished and often replaced by hypotonia of the muscle.

That is, the disturbance of muscle tone we call rigidity is actually overcorrected! The patient whose muscles are hypotonic looks "loose jointed" in bodily movements. The anticholinergic drugs can also alleviate rigidity, but rarely to the point of hypotonia.

Tremor is greatly reduced and often abolished by drug treatment. Of course, even if tremor is reduced by 80% or so, there is still some tremor and so the effect of treatment is not always fully appreciated. All the anti-Parkinson drugs relieve tremor to some extent. Sedative drugs also alleviate tremor but to a lesser extent and only at the expense of some drowsiness. Levodopa sometimes *increases* the tremor of Parkinson's disease at the outset of therapy, but on continued treatment it relieves the tremor more effectively than any other drug available today.

Bradykinesia, or akinesia, is reduced by all the drugs, and when mild or moderate it is usually abolished completely; however, when severe, it may be only partially reduced. In patients with severe parkinsonism, akinesia is the most distressing persistent symptom. In these cases, rigidity is abolished. Very little tremor is left, but significant akinesia may persist. Sometimes akinesia reappears briefly for a few minutes or so without tremor or rigidity.

Drug treatment can restore the automatic associated movements— eye blink, swallowing, swing of the arms while walking, expressive gestures, facial expressive movements, etc.—to normal or near normal. The amplitude of the voice and modulation of speech is improved. Disturbances of gait are also improved. The step becomes brisker, and the ability to walk slowly or rapidly and to turn around briskly can be restored. Shuffling, festination, and propulsion can be greatly diminished or completely abolished.

Feelings of numbness, weakness, aching or pulling pains, tightness, etc. are relieved. The excessive sweating and oiliness of the skin are also diminished. Pooling of saliva and drooling are greatly ameliorated. Painful cramps and the rare heat sensations called "thermal paresthesia" tend to be diminished but sometimes persist despite good treatment.

Change of medication may result in less effective control of the symptoms if one changes from a more-potent drug to a weaker one.

The re-emerging symptoms are sometimes interpreted as side effects. The patient thinks the new drug *caused* a feeling of weakness or dizziness or lethargy when in fact these are symptoms of the disease. In such circumstances, increasing the dose of the new drug often relieves these symptoms. This happens because it is difficult to judge the exact equivalent dose of the new drug which will give the same degree of anti-Parkinson effect. The doctor usually prefers to take the more conservative course; that is, changing over initially to a dose that is slightly less than the presumed equivalent dose in order to observe the patient's response, and then later to increase the dose as needed.

Because the disease continues to progress despite the best treatment possible, symptoms once well controlled may re-emerge or new symptoms may develop in the course of time. For example, a patient who had only mild tremor and rigidity on one side when the diagnosis of Parkinson's disease was made and treatment first begun may several years later experience some intermittent reappearance of the same tremor; or he may have a new symptom, such as a tendency to drag one foot while walking at times. In these circumstances patients often ask if the drug has lost its effect or if they themselves have become "resistant" to the drugs. Chances are it is merely a question of gradual progression of the disease, and a slight increase in dosage will probably control the symptoms again. Sometimes a change in activity or diet may alter the metabolism of the drugs and render a previously effective dose less effective. L-DOPA is especially sensitive to changes in eating habits. Its absorption may be delayed by foods rich in protein and by high-dosage vitamins. Thus if there has been a sudden loss of benefit from an effective drug regimen, it is a good idea to check for recent changes in diet, life style, or activity, or if the change coincides with the introduction of a new drug or vitamin supplements.

Whereas some patients require increases in the dosage over the years, others develop an increased sensitivity. To keep the effect the same, they must take smaller doses. It is thus possible for a new symptom to represent a side effect rather than a manifestation of the disease. In case of doubt, it is usually best to lower the dose slightly and watch what happens. If the new symptom is a side effect, it should diminish. If, on the other hand, the new symptom is in fact an expression of the disease, it should become more prominent. If the patient has been following a well-defined, regular schedule of medication, it is then a simple matter to make appropriate adjustments to find the optimal dose.

Sometimes the drugs produce results opposite to those expected. Whereas they relieve symptoms at one dose, they may increase certain symptoms at a higher dose. This is called a "paradoxical" effect. One of my patients, Mr. O., was troubled chiefly by a slowness of movement and stiffness in his legs while walking when I first saw him. Treatment with L-DOPA improved these symptoms to a moderate degree at the modest dose of 4 grams of L-DOPA daily. I directed Mr. O. and his wife to increase the dose gradually to 5 grams and then to 6 grams daily, but he failed to improve further. In fact, Mrs. O. reported that at a higher dose he was actually slower and stiffer. When Mr. O. discontinued his medication for several days for a religious fast, he reported that he actually felt better. He then remained off his medication completely for several more days. Although he felt better at first, he gradually became worse again and all his original symptoms returned. He then resumed taking L-DOPA and found that he felt best at a daily dose of 3 grams. Puzzled by this observation, I admitted Mr. O. to the hospital to study his reaction to L-DOPA more objectively. He was treated with a very small dose of L-DOPA for several days, then with a full dose for several days. He was examined hourly during the day, and blood samples were taken to measure the amount of DOPA. When the results were in, it was clear that Mr. O. did indeed have a striking paradoxical response to L-DOPA treatment. The higher the dose and the higher the blood level, the greater were his symptoms: He was slower and walked more stiffly. When he set out to walk, his feet seemed to hesitate as if his shoes were momentarily stuck to the floor. This curious phenomenon has been called "start hesitation" and has been observed as a paradoxical effect in occasional patients on higher doses.

Thus if a new symptom appears after an increase in the dose, the possibility of a paradoxical response should be considered. In such circumstances, there may be a narrow range over which the dosage is optimal. Going above or below that range makes matters worse! Finding the optimal dose may require considerable patience and care in making dosage adjustments. It requires close cooperation of patient and doctor.

DRUG HOLIDAYS

It was first noted some years ago by Dr. Richard Sweet at the New York Hospital, that when L-DOPA therapy was withdrawn for 1 week or more, and then resumed, it was more effective for a time. This observation was soon confirmed by others and led to the widespread use of "drug holidays" in the hope of restoring responsiveness to L-DOPA. With further experience, the "drug holiday" has proved useful chiefly in managing chronic L-DOPA overdosage with severe involuntary movements and mental disturbances. It may be a difficult, unpleasant, even dangerous experience for the patient, and should be done only by a physician experienced in its use, preferably in the hospital.

CHAPTER 6

Anticholinergic Drugs

The first type of drug a parkinsonian patient is likely to be given by his doctor is an anticholinergic agent of some kind. Most patients continue to take an anticholinergic drug for many years, even when levodopa or other drugs are also prescribed. There are a considerable number of anticholinergic agents, but since their effects are virtually identical they may be considered together as a group. Members of this large class of useful drugs were the first effective agents used in the treatment of parkinsonism.

The first anticholinergics were derived from plants. Just how they came to be used in treating parkinsonism is not clear. The first definite mention of their use for this purpose seems to be a comment in a doctoral thesis dated 1869 by a medical student in Paris that Professor Charcot was then administering some hyoscine to patients with Parkinson's disease at the Sâlpétrière, the old city hospital of Paris for chronic invalids. Hyoscine, also called scopolamine, is the active ingredient of the plant *Datura stramonium*, known popularly as jimsonweed or thorn apple. Wine extracts of the plant had been used for centuries as tincture of stramonium in the treatment of stomach cramps and abdominal colic. Closely related botanical preparations are the alcoholic extracts or "tincture" of the plant *Hyoscyamus niger* (black henbane) and the extract of *Atropa belladona* (deadly nightshade). The active principles are named hyoscyamine and atropine, respectively. The plants are members of the potato

69

family, called Solanaceae in botanical terminology. The extracts are alkaline and bitter tasting; hence they are termed "solanaceous alkaloids."

Tincture of belladonna as well as its active ingredients, or "principles," atropine and hyoscine (scopolamine) are still important drugs in medical practice. Their value was known in ancient times, and their present day uses were well established long before their mechanism of action was understood. It is now known that they act on the vagus nerve, which controls the stomach, intestine, bladder, and heart. The vagus nerve transmits its influence to the various organs through the action of a chemical intermediary, or messenger. The chemical nature of this messenger substance was identified over 40 years ago. It was called acetylcholine. The solanaceous alkaloids work by blocking the action of acetylcholine and hence are classed as anticholinergic drugs.

The various preparations of the potato plant drugs (or, more properly, solanaceous alkaloids) were the main form of drug treatment of parkinsonism for nearly 100 years. Various preparations were favored at one time or another. For example, for a time during the 1930s atropine preparations made from belladonna plants grown in Bulgaria enjoyed a reputation of being superior to other preparations although no explanation for this was apparent. Later, during the 1940s, a tablet containing a mixture of the three alkaloids marketed under the name Rabellon was very popular in the treatment of parkinsonism.

For some unknown reason, patients with postencephalitic parkinsonism tolerate much larger doses of anticholinergic drugs than can normal people or even patients with Parkinson's disease. The postencephalitic cases were also quite numerous during the 1920s and 1930s, and thus particular attention was directed to their treatment. Various regimens of treatment with the solanaceous alkaloids were developed, such as Roemer's high-dosage atropine treatment in which doses which would today be considered fantastic were routinely employed. The results were much more impressive in the postencephalitic cases than in the Parkinson's disease patients.

The high dosages of the drugs used produced side effects including mental confusion, mild incoordination, slurred speech, and forgetfulness, which collectively were known as the "belladonna jag." Similar symptoms of anticholinergic intoxication may occur in Parkinson's disease patients with much smaller doses. Other side effects included blurring of vision, dryness of the mouth, loss of sweating, and constipation.

SYNTHETIC ANTICHOLINERGICS

Once the chemical structure of acetylcholine was known, chemists were able to synthesize new chemical compounds in the laboratory to imitate or block its action. Thus synthetic anticholinergic drugs were developed which, it was hoped, would be more effective than the natural drugs derived from the potato plants. One of the first of these drugs was marketed under the name caramiphen (Panparnit). It was widely used as an anti-Parkinson agent for a time but is now no longer available. It was followed by the drug trihexyphenidyl (Artane), which was introduced as an anti-Parkinson drug by the late Dr. Doshay, Dr. Schwab of Boston, and others during the years 1949–1951. It appeared to have fewer side effects than the older potato plant drugs and to be equally effective. Trihexyphenidyl has been and is still widely used in the treatment of parkinsonism. It was rapidly followed by three other closely related drugs: procyclidine (Kemadrin), cycrimine (Pagitane), and biperiden (Akineton). Trihexyphenidyl is also marketed as Tremin and as Pipanol by other manufacturers.

Trihexyphenidyl and its three cousins are very similar. In fact, in their clinical effects they are quite indistinguishable and can be used interchangeably. For most of the 20 years from 1950 to 1970 (that is, until the introduction of levodopa), these were the chief anti-Parkinson drugs in common use. They are still important drugs and are useful in the initial treatment of mild cases of parkinsonism or as an adjunct to levodopa therapy. They are also useful in treating drug-induced parkinsonism as well. In contrast to levodopa, these drugs can reverse the parkinsonism induced by tranquilizer drugs.

Trihexyphenidyl is available in white 2- and 5-mg scored tablets and in a blue 5-mg slow-release capsule. The normal starting dose is one 2-mg tablet three times daily. For patients who are sensitive to the side effects of anticholinergic drugs, the 2-mg scored tablet may be broken in half and 1 mg taken two or three times daily. If the 2-mg tablet is well tolerated, the dose may be increased to one 5-mg tablet three times daily. More than 15 mg daily is rarely helpful in Parkinson's disease. Indeed, most patients cannot tolerate large doses. However, postencephalitic cases may tolerate and require much larger doses. I know some postencephalitic patients who take up to 40 to 50 mg of this drug daily with excellent benefit and no side effects.

Another synthetic anticholinergic agent widely used in treating parkinsonism is benztropine mesylate (Cogentin). The molecular structure of this drug is closely patterned after that of atropine; hence, the "tropine" in its generic name. It is somewhat more potent than trihexyphenidyl and is consequently made in smaller dosage forms: 1- and 2-mg tablets. The latter is scored so that the tablet can be broken into four equal parts. A patient can thus be given 0.5 mg per dose. It is also available, as is biperiden (Akineton), in a liquid form for injection with a hypodermic needle. It is used to treat parkinsonism and other similar reactions to tranquilizer drugs. A single injection can terminate the tranquilizer reaction within minutes.

A small group of anticholinergic drugs which are no longer widely used are, strangely enough, close cousins to the major tranquilizers. They include ethopropazine (Parsidol) and diethazine (Diparcol). Only ethopropazine is available in the United States. Diethazine was withdrawn because of some serious adverse reactions but is still used in most other countries. Ethopropazine is made in the form of 50- and 100-mg white tablets. The usual dose is one 100-mg tablet three or four times daily.

ANTIHISTAMINES

Atropine was widely used in the treatment of asthma until fairly recently. The search for a drug which would have atropine's effect in asthma and other allergies led to the development of the drug diphenhydramine (Benadryl). The success of this new drug, introduced around 1946, resulted in the introduction of many related drugs for the treatment of allergies. Their beneficial effect is thought to be due to their ability to block the action of the natural substance histamine formed in the body during allergic reactions; these drugs are thus classified as *antihistamines*. Some of the drugs, notably diphenhydramine, were accidentally found to have some effect on the symptoms of Parkinson's disease. Two drugs of this class have been marketed specifically for use in treating parkinsonism: orphenadrine hydrochloride (Disipal) and chlorophenoxamine (Phenoxene). Although diphenhydramine itself has not been marketed and advertised to physicians as an anti-Parkinson drug, it has been widely used in treating parkinsonism. The dosage of these drugs required to affect parkinsonian symptoms is 50 mg two to four times daily.

Many other antihistamines not normally thought of as anti-Parkinson drugs nevertheless affect parkinsonian symptoms. The reason antihistamines may be helpful in parkinsonism has nothing to do with their properties as antihistamines but with the fact that all have some anticholinergic properties. Trihexyphenidyl is approximately 25 times more potent an anticholinergic agent than is diphenhydramine, and so the latter is used in dosages 25 times as great. Thus 50 mg of diphenhydramine is as effective in relieving parkinsonian symptoms as 2 mg of trihexyphenidyl. Indeed, it appears that any drug having some anticholinergic effect also has some anti-Parkinson effect.

There are drugs which enhance or imitate the action in the nervous system of the chemical messenger acetylcholine. These are, naturally, called "cholinergic" drugs. It is an interesting fact that cholinergic drugs exacerbate the symptoms of parkinsonism! For example, injection of a small dose of the drug physostigmine (which enhances the action of acetylcholine in the brain) produces within minutes a marked increase in the tremor, rigidity, and other symptoms of parkinsonism. This effect can be promptly canceled by an injection of scopolamine or benztropine (Cogentin); if left alone, the effect subsides spontaneously within approximately 45 minutes.

It is clearly a good idea for Parkinson patients to avoid cholinergic drugs. In practice, however, very few cholinergic drugs are used, and the likelihood of a patient encountering one inadvertently (that is, one that can get into the brain and exacerbate the parkinsonian symptoms) is quite remote. Only two cholinergic drugs are used at all extensively in medical practice: pilocarpine, which is used in the form of eyedrops to treat glaucoma, and bethanecol (Urecholine), which is used to stimulate the bladder. These drugs do not affect parkinsonian symptoms. The manufacturer of bethanecol lists parkinsonism in the prescribing directions as a condition in which this drug should not be used. However, I have often used it to stimulate sluggish bladders of Parkinson patients and have never seen an adverse effect on the parkinsonian symptoms. It is highly unlikely that bethanecol in the doses ordinarily used can have an effect on the Parkinson state.

ANTICHOLINERGIC DRUG INTOXICATION

All the drugs discussed so far depend for their usefulness in treating parkinsonism on the fact that they are anticholinergic. That is, that they block the action of the chemical messenger acetylcholine in the brain. By the same token, their side effects are due to the same mechanism. Blocking acetylcholine too severely produces undesirable effects, and the side effects are essentially the same with all of the anticholinergic drugs. There is a common pattern which we term "anticholinergic intoxication."

The most common side effects are dryness of the mouth, blurring of near vision, constipation, and weakening of the bladder. In addition, there is a whole range of mental side effects.

Dryness of the mouth is due to a reduced flow of saliva. The saliva is also thicker and harder to swallow. The throat and nose may feel dry. The symptom is most marked when first starting treatment with anticholinergics. Partial tolerance develops within a few weeks, and most patients find it only a minor nuisance on continuing treatment. Some seek relief by sucking on bitter lemon candies or other hard sweets.

Blurring of near vision is due to the fact that anticholinergic drugs tend to diminish the action of the fine muscle in the eye, which changes the shape of the lens to focus on near objects. Normally the eye has universal focus for everything more than 18 inches away. To get a sharp view of objects which are closer, it is necessary to change the shape of the lens of the eye. This change is called "accommodation." The eye doctor regularly puts drops of atropine or a synthetic anticholinergic in the eye for the purpose of "paralyzing accommodation" so that the optical properties of the eye can be tested precisely. Taking an anticholinergic drug by mouth produces the same effect, but to a lesser degree. For this reason many patients notice difficulty in reading or doing close work when they first start on anticholinergic drugs. People normally have increasing difficulty with near vision after reaching middle age, called *presbyopia*. Age renders the individual more susceptible to this effect of anticholinergics. In addition, anticholinergics cause the pupil to open a bit more widely. This may also contribute to the blurring of near vision. Generally, the visual effect of the anticholinergics diminishes after awhile. If it proves persistent, however, a new set of reading glasses can be obtained.

The tendency to widen or dilate the pupil may exacerbate glaucoma. Patients who have Parkinson's disease and glaucoma should be carefully checked by their eye doctor when treatment with anticholinergics is begun. If the glaucoma is under proper treatment or has been surgically corrected, there is usually no difficulty. The eye doctor can readily check the pressure of the eye to make sure that the treatment for the parkinsonism does not adversely affect the glaucoma.

Anticholinergic drugs typically slow the motor activity of the intestine. The waves of contraction called peristalsis are slowed. It is for this reason that many anticholinergic drugs are employed for the treatment of disorders of the stomach and intestine. However, by the same token, the constipation of Parkinson's disease may be somewhat increased. This is rarely a serious problem, but if constipation is troublesome, it can be managed with gentle laxatives.

A similar calming effect is exerted by anticholinergic drugs on the musculature of the urinary bladder. In a sense, these drugs sedate the bladder. This may be helpful to the patient who is troubled with urinary urgency and a need to get up several times during the night to void. An anticholinergic drug given at bedtime may help relieve this symptom. However, in the older male patient who has trouble due to an enlarged prostate gland obstructing the flow of urine, this calming effect can lead to urinary retention. Thus anticholinergic drugs are given with caution to patients who have symptoms of prostatic obstruction. The need to pass a catheter can usually be averted by using very small doses of the drug. It may, of course, be necessary to operate on the prostate. A specialist in urology should be consulted before symptoms of urinary obstruction reach a severe stage.

The mental effects of anticholinergic drugs are important and, in many ways, very interesting. The fact that ingestion of the leaves of *Datura stramonium* (jimsonweed), henbane, or deadly nightshade can cause mental disturbances has been known since ancient times. Abuse of these botanicals for psychedelic effects has been described repeatedly. Every year or two I read a report of another case of poisoning in a child who has eaten leaves of jimsonweed. The symptoms include confusion, agitation, hallucinations, stupor, and, in severe intoxication, coma. The symptoms subside within a day or two except for amnesia for the episode.

The first and commonest mental side effect noticeable in patients on treatment with any anticholinergic drug is forgetfulness, mainly for recent events. The patient may forget where he left his glasses a minute ago or fails to remember what he went to the corner store to buy. Occasional mild confusion then appears. Visual illusions are especially frequent. Familiar objects may be mistaken for something else. The patient may mention seeing worms on the floor, whereas actually there is a design in the flooring which is misinterpreted because the pattern seems to move. Spectral illusions generally of a benign if not pleasing character are experienced. There may be hallucinations of people or animals roaming about the house. Most commonly, there seem to be complex scenes with a group of people wandering about, having a party. They may be smaller than normal and seem to go about their business without disturbing the patient. Patients may experience these visions for long periods of time but are afraid to mention them to anyone for fear of being thought "crazy." Finally, however, in a moment of confusion, the patient reacts to these illusions. Some patients angrily order the strangers out of the house, accuse them of stealing, or call the police to chase them away. At this point, the patient's family, not having previously noticed anything out of the ordinary, becomes alarmed. There is, however, no reason to be frightened. These disturbances disappear if the dosage of the anticholinergic drug is reduced. The physician should check to see if these disturbances followed a change in medication or the addition of a new drug. A patient who has been doing well on a standard dose of, say, trihexyphenidyl may suddenly develop such mental disturbances when another drug is added. For example, the patient may have taken an antihistamine because of hayfever symptoms. The anticholinergic properties of the antihistamine *added to* the anticholinergic properties of trihexyphenidyl then carried the patient over the threshold into a mild state of anticholinergic intoxication. Usually the disturbance subsides within a day or so after the new drug is discontinued. If there has been no change of medication, the patient's drug regimen may be revised downward. Usually it is not a good idea to give a tranquilizer unless there is severe agitation. Many of the commonly used major tranquilizers also have some anticholinergic properties, and so the confusion and hallucinations may be increased even if the agitation is controlled for a few hours.

Some patients are very sensitive to the toxic mental effects of the anticholinergic drugs and cannot tolerate any of these drugs, not even very mild ones such as the antihistamines. A few patients develop these mental reactions after even the mildest sleep medications. Rarely, a patient experiences these disturbances spontaneously, on no treatment at all. There is probably something inherent to Parkinson's disease which makes one prone to develop these mental disturbances.

Another effect of the anticholinergic drugs that may be good or bad, depending on the circumstances, is the tendency to reduce sweating. Excessive sweating, sometimes occurring irregularly in bursts, is an occasional symptom of Parkinson's disease. Anticholinergic drugs can diminish this excessive perspiration—sometimes not as much as desired and sometimes too much. We depend on sweating to cool our bodies in warm weather. The brain controls the amount of sweat we produce, thereby regulating body temperature. Anticholinergic drugs may impair this regulation, and in warm weather fever and even coma may result. This is a rare occurrence today but was a familiar problem years ago when large doses of atropine were commonly used in treating parkinsonism.

ADVERSE REACTIONS

Adverse reactions have been very rare with the anticholinergic drugs. I have never seen one, but there are reports in medical journals of isolated instances of allergic skin rashes, inflammation of the liver, and a rare toxic effect on the bone marrow resulting in a lack of white blood corpuscles. The last-mentioned condition is very dangerous and potentially lethal. Most of the cases reported occurred with the drug diethazine (Diparcol), which is used infrequently today and is no longer available in the United States.

AMANTADINE

A Parkinson patient of the late Dr. Schwab reported that while taking the drug amantadine as protection against catching the flu she felt better. This drug had been developed as an antiviral agent and is protective against the flu virus. Dr. Schwab confirmed this observation and then treated other Parkinson patients with amantadine, finding that many of these patients looked and felt better while taking the drug. Other doctors also tried amantadine in their Parkinson patients and corroborated Dr. Schwab's report.

Amantadine does indeed possess some property that partially alleviates the symptoms of Parkinson's disease. How it does so and what this property may be is not known. The side effects—blurring of vision, constipation, mental confusion, dryness of the mouth—suggest that it acts as an anticholinergic drug. However, laboratory studies have thus far failed to show any acetylcholine blocking effect. Some scientists have reported that amantadine enhances the function of dopamine nerve cells. However, this effect has only been shown *in vitro*, with amounts of the drug far greater than the dosages that can be used in humans. Thus, although it is often listed as a "dopaminergic" drug, I do not agree that amantadine can be so classified.

Amantadine (Symmetrel) is available in a 100-mg red capsule. The normal dose is one capsule two or three times daily, although some patients may take as many as four. Since it may augment the side effects of anticholinergic drugs such as trihexyphenidyl, care is usually taken to change doses slowly when using the two drugs simultaneously.

A unique and unusual side effect of amantadine is the appearance of a curious faint purplish mottling of the skin of the legs and sometimes the arms due to blood pooling in small veins in the skin. It usually appears only after several months and may take 1 to 2 months to subside after the drug is stopped. This unusual side effect is apparently harmless. It is called livido reticularis (Fig. 8). When I see it in a new patient, I can surmise with some confidence that the patient has probably been taking amantadine. Sometimes the purplish mottling is accompanied by swelling of the feet and ankles due to the accumulation of water in the soft tissues. The medical term for this accumulation of water is *edema*. Although it may be ungainly and worrisome, this too appears to be harmless and disappears when amantadine is discontinued.

Another curious property of amantadine is that it may lose its effectiveness after several months. However, if the patient stops taking the drug for awhile and then uses it again, it usually regains its effectiveness. Although this phenomenon occurs in only some patients, it is still worthwhile when a patient has been taking amantadine for some time, to determine if it is still effective. I often advise my patients in such circumstances to discontinue the drug

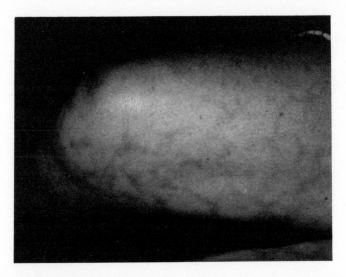

FIG. 8. Livido reticularis, the purplish mottling of the skin on the leg of a patient treated with amantadine.

for a week or so. If there is no change and the patient does not feel worse, there seems no point in taking it again. It may then be discontinued completely and tried again after a month or two. If, on the other hand, the patient is definitely worse after stopping the amantadine, the drug treatment should be promptly resumed since it is clear that the drug is worth taking.

CHAPTER 7

From L-DOPA to Levodopa

L-DOPA is the most effective substance currently available for the
treatment of Parkinson's disease. Its full chemical name is L-3,4-
dihydroxyphenylalanine. Chemists have for many years abbreviated
this cumbersome name to the simpler "DOPA" or "L-DOPA." Persons not versed in the language of chemistry sometimes fear that
the name DOPA has a more sinister meaning. Patients often ask if
the drug L-DOPA contains "dope." Many wonder if it is a Spanish
drug, for they understand L-DOPA to be *El Dopa*. Others inquire
about the ingredients of L-DOPA.

L-DOPA is in fact merely a simple chemical substance occurring
in nature in both animals and plants. It is not a mixture of ingredients
but a single rather simple molecule belonging to a class of substances
known to chemists as *amino acids* and composed of atoms of carbon,
hydrogen, oxygen, and nitrogen. The arrangement of these atoms
in the DOPA molecule is shown in Fig. 9. Its shape in three-
dimensional space is such that the DOPA molecule can exist in two
forms, each the mirror image of the other, just as the right hand is
the mirror image of the left. The bones and ligaments of both hands
are connected in exactly the same way, yet the two hands are not
exactly the same in three-dimensional space; they cannot fit in the
same glove. The two forms of the DOPA molecule are designated
the *levo* form (from the Latin *laevo*, meaning left) and the *dextro*

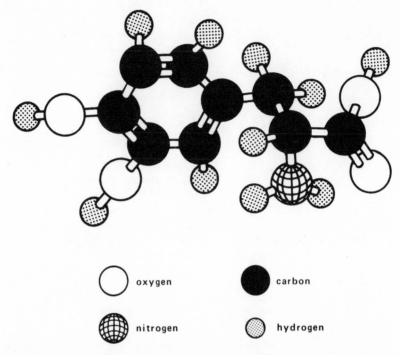

FIG. 9. Model of the DOPA molecule. The nitrogen and its attached hydrogen atoms form an *amine* group, which confers on the molecule the chemical properties of an alkali. The group at the far right end of the molecule—consisting of a carbon atom holding an oxygen atom with two arms or *bonds* and an oxygen-hydrogen combination with another bond—is called a *carboxyl* group; it confers on the molecule the properties of an acid. DOPA is thus an *amino acid*. Removal of the carboxyl group—a step called *decarboxylation* and controlled by an enzyme aptly enough called a *decarboxylase*—converts the DOPA molecule to a dopamine molecule.

form (from the Latin prefix *dexter*, meaning right)—or more simply, the L- and D-forms.

Many molecules exist in duplicate mirror forms, such as L-glucose and D-glucose, L-amphetamine and D-amphetamine, L-tryptophan and D-tryptophan, and so on. Just as your right hand cannot fit in a left-hand glove, so the L-forms of these molecules cannot fit in the same spaces as the D-forms. Consequently, the two forms of these molecules often have different physical properties, form crystals of different shapes, and behave differently in the biological world. It is a remarkable fact that plants and animals make and use only the L-forms! Only the L-form of dopa is found in nature, and only the L-form is effective in treating Parkinson's disease. The D-form is inert!

L-DOPA was first discovered over 70 years ago in the broad bean or "fava" bean *(Vicia fava)* used in Mediterranean cooking. It is also present in the velvet bean *(Mucuna pruriens)*, the "loco weed," and certain other related legumes. Botanists have suggested that L-DOPA serves to protect the plants from insects.

L-DOPA also occurs in the animal kingdom, where it plays an important role as an intermediate substance in the metabolism of adrenaline, the hormone secreted into the circulation by the adrenal gland to prepare the body for "fight or flight" in an emergency. The adrenal gland makes adrenaline in a series of chemical reactions that begin with the amino acid *tyrosine*, an ingredient of our diet. Tyrosine is found mainly in the proteins we eat every day. An ordinary American hamburger, for example, contains 1 to 2 grams of tyrosine. When we eat a hamburger or other meat, during the process of digestion the protein molecules are broken down to simpler molecules called peptides. These in turn are broken down further into their component amino acids, which are then absorbed by the intestines and transported in the blood first to the liver and then to other organs throughout the body. Most of the tyrosine we absorb from our daily diet is used to build new protein. A very small proportion is taken up from the circulation by the cells of the adrenal gland. There it is immediately converted by a single molecular rearrangement to form the amino acid L-DOPA. L-DOPA in turn is promptly changed into dopamine via another chemical reaction. In turn, dopamine is changed into norepinephrine, and in the final step in this metabolic pathway noradrenaline is converted into adrenaline. The adrenaline is then stored by the cells of the adrenal gland in little packets, which can be seen under the electron microscope, until such time as the gland receives a signal from the nervous system to release it into the bloodstream.

This pathway of sequential chemical reactions occurs in exactly the same way in the substantia nigra of the brain. Here, however, the process ends with the formation of dopamine. The dopamine is then stored in these cells and their fibers, which spread throughout the corpus striatum, until released to function as a chemical messenger to other nerve cells. In other areas of the nervous system (for example, in the sympathetic nerves), the process ends with the formation of noradrenaline.

The step from tyrosine to DOPA in the adrenal gland and the brain is strictly controlled and is called a "rate-limiting" step. Feeding large amounts of tyrosine does not result in the formation of larger amounts of dopamine or of noradrenaline or adrenaline. This is not surprising. If it were not so, every time we ate a lot of protein we would have too much adrenaline in our systems. However, the step from L-DOPA to dopamine is not subject to such control, and so it is possible to increase the amount of dopamine formed in the brain by feeding large amounts of L-DOPA. Thus tyrosine has little effect in treating parkinsonism whereas L-DOPA is very effective. Essentially, L-DOPA relieves the symptoms of parkinsonism by restoring brain dopamine at least partially to normal levels. L-DOPA itself is inert. All of its actions are due to the dopamine derived from it in the various organs of the body.

L-DOPA is the name employed by chemists to describe this interesting substance. However, L-DOPA prepared for use as a drug is officially termed levodopa. This is the international generic name of the medicinal form of L-DOPA. It is marketed, of course, under various trade names by different pharmaceutical firms. In the United States it is made available by Hoffman LaRoche as Larodopa, and by Eaton Laboratories as Dopar. In the remainder of this book, I refer to it by its generic name levodopa.

Levodopa taken by mouth passes through the stomach into the duodenum and then to the upper and small intestine where it is absorbed. The process of absorption takes place over a period of several hours. We can study this process by measuring (via chemical means) the amount of levodopa in the blood at various intervals after a dose is ingested. Measurements done on different patients or on the same patient on different days vary somewhat, but in general the level of levodopa in the blood (normally zero) gradually rises to a peak value approximately 2 to 3 hours after a dose is taken by mouth, then gradually falls back to zero again within 4 to 6 hours. The results of such a study, plotted as a graph, are seen in Fig. 10.

From such studies, a number of things have been found to influence the absorption of levodopa. One of the most important is the amount and type of food in the stomach. Solid food, especially food containing protein, delays the absorption of levodopa and may reduce the amount taken up in the circulation. Many patients are aware

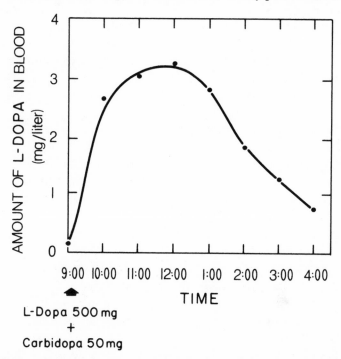

FIG. 10. Graph shows the amount of levodopa at various times in the blood of a patient after a single dose was administered at 9:00 A.M. Blood was then drawn from a vein each hour until 4:00 P.M. The highest blood level of levodopa was measured in the sample taken at 12:00 noon.

of this effect of food. They have observed that the relief of their symptoms is greater and comes on more rapidly when they take a dose of levodopa on an empty stomach than when they take it after a meal. Many have also noted that their usual dose may have little or no effect if taken after a hearty steak dinner. Patients on a low-protein diet need less levodopa to obtain the same result they experience with higher doses on a regular diet.

If the stomach is excessively acid, it empties into the duodenum more slowly, and consequently the absorption of levodopa is delayed. In such circumstances, taking some milk or an antacid tablet with the levodopa improves the absorption of levodopa. Some patients have noted that chewing the levodopa tablet rather than swallowing it provides faster relief of their symptoms. They use this trick for a "booster" effect usually with supplementary midafternoon doses.

Once absorbed into the circulation, levodopa travels throughout the entire body. A large proportion of the dose taken by mouth ends up in muscles, fat stores, the liver, skin, kidney, and other organs. Most of it is rapidly converted to dopamine in the blood vessels in the various organs, especially the kidney, and is excreted in the urine in the form of various inactive substances.

Only a very small proportion of the oral dose of levodopa, probably less than 1%, ultimately penetrates the brain. There it is selectively taken up by the dopamine nerve cells of the substantia nigra and possibly also by the other cells and then converted to dopamine. In this manner the brain stores of dopamine may be at least partially replenished.

Of course, some time is required for the levodopa to leave the bloodstream, cross the walls of the blood vessels, enter the brain, and reach the dopamine cells, where it may then be converted to dopamine. Animal studies indicate that this delay is of the order of 15 to 30 minutes. Thus if the peak blood level of levodopa is reached 2 hours after ingestion, the peak brain level of dopamine must be reached at approximately 2 hours 15 minutes to 2 hours 30 minutes after ingestion. Of course, some effects may begin to be felt 20 to 30 minutes after taking a dose of levodopa by mouth, but the full effect does not occur until at least 2 hours later. The newly formed dopamine in the brain joins the dopamine formed in the normal manner from tyrosine as just described. In this way, brain dopamine stores are replenished and the symptoms of parkinsonism are correspondingly diminished.

Levodopa treatment, however, is not a cure. So far as we know it does not affect the basic disease process—whatever it may be—responsible for the dysfunction of the brain's dopamine cells or bring back those that may have deteriorated. It merely helps the dopamine nerve cells make dopamine more readily. Apparently it helps the cells function better despite their illness. Levodopa treatment is thus a *symptomatic* treatment. That is, it is a treatment that can relieve symptoms without correcting the underlying or primary cause. It may also be considered a replacement therapy—that is, a treatment based on replacing a substance essential to the body's economy that is deficient. The same may be said of other forms of treatment in modern medicine: thyroid hormone treatment for hypothyroidism, for example, or insulin treatment for diabetes. In diabetes mellitus there is a deficiency of insulin, the hormone that regulates sugar metabolism throughout the body. The diabetic patient may be given insulin by injection to provide the body with the insulin it needs but for some reason is unable to make itself in sufficient amounts. In this way the disturbance in sugar metabolism which causes so much of the trouble in diabetes can be corrected. However, insulin does not cure diabetes. It does not correct the basic disease—whatever it is—and restore to the body the ability to make proper amounts of insulin.

When levodopa treatment is first begun, the patient feels a gradual improvement over a period of several days. An appreciable response is usually achieved within 3 to 5 days, but still further improvement builds up more slowly over the subsequent weeks. The full effect of treatment may not be apparent for 2 to 3 months of continuing treatment. Most patients are not aware of the effect of each individual dose. Nor are they aware of any definite change if they miss a given dose. If a dose is missed inadvertently, there is little point in trying to make up the lost dose by taking more pills the next time the medicine is due. When treatment is stopped for any reason, the parkinsonian symptoms return gradually over a period of several days. Little change may be noted the first day. Definite change is experienced the second day after stopping treatment and still more the third and fourth days. Most of the benefit of levodopa treatment is lost by the fourth or fifth days, but it may take 1 to 2 weeks before the effect of levodopa is completely gone. The slowness of the response to treatment and the long duration of the response when treatment is stopped indicate that in most patients the brain is able to store dopamine for some period of time, and that to fill up the dopamine stores may require several months of continuing treatment. It is as if a large reservoir is being filled through a small opening with a small bucket. Many buckets and some time are required to fill the reservoir to its full capacity.

A few patients feel the effect of each dose of levodopa. They can tell when a given dose begins to work, to diminish their symptoms. They can also tell when the effect of a given dose wears off. Such patients may also experience some return of their parkinsonian symptoms in the morning, before the first dose of the day. They seem to have lost the "sleep benefit" which most patients have. Apparently the levodopa effect wears off overnight presumably because the dopamine reserves diminished during the long interval between the last dose at night and the first dose the following morning. In other words, these patients do not have a sufficiently good long-duration response to levodopa to maintain full control of their symptoms for a long time. They are said to have primarily a short-duration response. It is presumed that the lack of a long-duration response reflects decreased capacity to store dopamine. The reservoir is leaky, or it has become smaller.

In a small percentage of patients the response to levodopa appears to be chiefly of the short-duration variety. These patients fluctuate markedly from a state of parkinsonism to a state of normal movement and back again several times a day. The change from one state to the other may take place quite rapidly. Some patients have said that it felt as if an electric switch had been turned on or off. For this reason this phenomenon has been termed the *on-off effect*. The fluctuations can be smoothed out to some extent by adjusting the dosage schedule to the duration of the individual patient's response. Thus instead of taking levodopa only three or four times daily as is usual, such a patient might take it every 3 hours or even every 2 hours through the day. The precise timing can be very important and must be carefully worked out, by trial and error, in each patient. Generally results are best if the patient follows a definite schedule strictly "by the clock" and works closely with the doctor to develop the schedule which seems best suited. It is rarely worthwhile to take levodopa more frequently than every 2 hours. Some patients with this "on-off" problem are able to judge sufficiently in advance that an "off" phase is coming and so take their levodopa dose when they feel the need. However, in my experience most patients who self-regulate their dosage schedules depending on their own subjective feeling do poorly. They tend to overdose themselves and become confused about how much to take and when to take it. Often they cannot tell whether their symptoms at any one time are due to overdosage or underdosage, and fail to distinguish the symptoms of parkinsonism from the side effects of levodopa.

NAUSEA AND VOMITING

Dopamine formed from the levodopa the Parkinson patient takes by mouth accumulates not only in the striatum but in other brain areas as well. This may be all to the good, but it may also give rise to undesired or "side" effects. A major side effect in the early days when levodopa therapy was first being developed was nausea and vomiting. We have since learned to cope with this side effect, and it is no longer the problem it was. Moreover, levodopa is now usually given in combination with an enzyme inhibitor drug, either carbidopa or bensarizide, which prevents the conversion of levodopa to dopamine throughout the body *except* in the brain. A major benefit of this combination treatment is a marked decrease in the frequency and severity of nausea and vomiting. Nevertheless, since nausea and vomiting still occasionally occur even with the combination treatment, we should consider in some detail the mechanism of this unpleasant side effect before discussing the enzyme inhibitor drugs.

There is a specialized area located in the brainstem (shown schematically in Fig. 2, p. 4) near the junction of the brain and the spinal cord known as the area postrema. Here is the vomiting center. It contains nerve cells whose task it is to detect toxins or poisons in the circulation and to prevent further absorption of such substances by provoking vomiting to empty the stomach and throw out the offending material.

The vomiting center is sensitive to levodopa, adrenaline and many other substances. Apparently it regards levodopa, an unusual substance to find in the circulation, as an offensive material to be thrown out. As the blood level of levodopa rises approximately 1 to 1½ hours after a dose, the vomiting center may be activated. It can also be activated when levodopa is given by direct injection into the bloodstream through a vein. The vomiting induced by levodopa is not due to irritation of the stomach itself, although to the patient who experiences it, it makes little practical difference. There is first a general discomfort, a sense of weakness, and a disinterest in eating food. If the activation is more marked, there is a metallic taste in the mouth, nausea, and dizziness. These symptoms may subside after a half-hour or so, especially if the patient lies down. If the activation is sufficient, vomiting occurs even if there is nothing in the stomach. The vomiting usually comes very suddenly and is very quickly over, and the patient usually feels better soon afterward.

Unfortunately, the dose of levodopa required to relieve the symptoms of parkinsonism is more than enough to activate the vomiting center in most persons. There are exceptions, of course. I have seen patients who took full doses of levodopa alone from the first day of treatment and never felt any nausea. They are exceptional. At the other extreme, there are patients who never tolerate full doses of levodopa and fail to develop tolerance even after many months. In the early experiments with levodopa, this state of affairs was a major obstacle to the development of an effective means of using levodopa to treat parkinsonism. However, two facts about the vomiting center make it possible to overcome this problem in most patients.

The first is that after repeated exposure to levodopa the vomiting center gradually becomes accustomed to its presence and no longer responds to it. The second is that the vomiting center is most likely to react when the blood level of DOPA is rising rapidly; that is, when the levodopa taken by mouth is absorbed especially well. Thus it is possible to "tame" the vomiting center by starting treatment with small doses of levodopa, and by taking levodopa only after meals to slow its absorption.

In practice, the major problem has been with breakfast. Many people do not eat much for breakfast—a glass of orange juice, a cup of coffee, and toast—which is not enough to slow the absorption of levodopa. In fact, the caffeine in the coffee may help levodopa activate the vomiting center.

Patients taking their first doses of levodopa after such a small breakfast or nonbreakfast, if you will, are especially apt to feel at least some nausea or loss of interest in food. As lunchtime rolls around a few hours later, they may still be disinclined to eat and thus content themselves with a cup of coffee for lunch. This time, the vomiting center, still disturbed by the morning dose of levodopa, may react more violently and vomiting results. The answers to this problem are threefold: (1) make sure that breakfast includes some solid food, preferably food containing protein; (2) change to de-caffeinated coffee or tea; and (3) if necessary, reduce the breakfast dose of levodopa. If the patient still reacts with nausea and vomiting after these measures have been tried, the doctor may prescribe some antivomiting drug. Unfortunately, the most effective antivomiting drugs antagonize levodopa. They not only block the activation of the vomiting center by levodopa, they also prevent the relief of parkinsonism. The doctor must then fall back on milder antivomiting drugs, which often do the trick. Such drugs include: diphenidol (Vontrol) and trimethobenzamide (Tigan). The old anti-Parkinson drugs such as trihexyphenidyl (Artane) and even the common anti-histamine drug diphenhydramine hydrochloride (Benadryl) also give some protection against the activation of the vomiting center. Thus,

when beginning levodopa treatment a patient already taking trihexyphenidyl, procyclidine (Kemadrin), benztropine mesylate (Cogentin), or a drug of that class will probably do better to continue
it during the initial period of levodopa treatment. The daily medication schedule may need to be adjusted so that both drugs are taken
together. Protection against the vomiting effect of levodopa is greater
if the protecting drug is taken *with* levodopa and *before* the nausea
and vomiting begin. When the feeling of nausea has developed, it
is too late to expect much benefit from the protecting drug.

The more slowly the dose of levodopa is raised, the less likely
it is that nausea and vomiting will occur. Normally, it seems to take
3 to 6 months to develop full tolerance to the action of levodopa
on the vomiting center. Thus the patient should not be in too great
a hurry to enjoy the good effects of levodopa in full measure. Both
patient and physician should be willing to wait a few months before
reaching the ultimate dosage schedule. Of course, personal tolerance
levels vary considerably. Some patients never experience even the
slightest nausea, whereas others are unable to develop a sufficient
tolerance to reach effective doses of levodopa even after several
years. Fortunately for the latter patients, activation of the vomiting
center can be prevented by the "inhibitor" drug carbidopa, which
is discussed in detail further on.

INVOLUNTARY MOVEMENTS

The most common side effect of levodopa treatment is the production of various involuntary movements. These include twitches,
jerks, nods, gestures, twisting or writhing movements, or simple
restlessness. The neurological term for these movements is *chorea*.
These movements can be so minimal as to be barely perceptible.
Only a relative or close friend who knows the patient can detect
them. When they are somewhat more obvious but still very mild,
they seem to be no more than restlessness or fidgetiness. Usually,
patients are not aware of them until they become at least mild in
magnitude. Patients usually do not mind the movements even when
they are quite obvious. When severe, they become tiring and cause
clumsiness and awkwardness.

The movements appear at higher doses and always disappear when the dosage of levodopa is reduced. In fact, they usually occur only for a brief period, 2 to 3 hours after the last daily dose of levodopa, a time when the brain levels of dopamine are highest.

The movements can be abolished by drugs that block the action of dopamine (for example, the major tranquilizers). However, these drugs also block the desired effects of levodopa and thus are useful only in emergency situations to treat overdosage with levodopa. Many treatments have been tried in the hope of finding a way of preventing the movements without also preventing the relief of parkinsonian symptoms. Thus far, no effective means of doing this has been found. The only way of handling the problem is to lower the dosage of levodopa until the movements cease. Unfortunately, many patients then have some recurrence of their parkinsonism. Most patients prefer a compromise in which some movements are present and better relief of the parkinsonism is obtained. In my experience, this dilemma is the major shortcoming of levodopa therapy.

In many ways, chorea and parkinsonism are "opposites." In chorea there is excessive bodily movement, whereas in parkinsonism there is too little bodily movement. In chorea the muscles are loose and floppy; in parkinsonism they are stiff and rigid. Drugs which cause parkinsonism are useful in treating chorea. It seems that, conversely, levodopa, a drug which can cause chorea, is useful in treating parkinsonism.

Thus the production of chorea-like movements in a Parkinson patient reflects an overcorrection of the parkinsonism and an excessive amount of dopamine in the brain at the precise moment the movements are present. A half-hour later, when the movements cease, it may be presumed that the brain dopamine level has decreased to a more desirable range.

Frankly, the involuntary chorea-like movements are not really a "side effect" in the sense of an adverse reaction but, rather, a normal effect of levodopa in Parkinson patients which, although undesirable, merely reflects the dosage. Curiously, levodopa does not so readily induce these involuntary movements in patients with other disorders or in normal volunteers. Parkinsonian patients are more susceptible to the chorea-inducing effect of levodopa than are other people. Other drugs which alleviate parkinsonism can also induce the involuntary movements, although to a lesser extent. Of course, these other drugs are also less effective in relieving the symptoms of parkinsonism. It seems, then, that the involuntary movements are due not only to the drug but also to something in the Parkinson brain. Just what that "something" may be is not known. It seems reasonable to suspect that certain changes which occur in the brain to compensate for the longstanding depletion of dopamine may be responsible.

The brain is somehow able to compensate for a great loss of dopamine for a very long time. How does it do this? One way seems to be to increase the rate at which dopamine is formed, perhaps to correct for the decreased capacity to store it. Another way the brain may compensate seems to be to increase its sensitivity to the actions of dopamine so that a smaller amount may provoke the same response. The brain cells which normally receive and respond to dopamine may thus become supersensitive to it and thereby adapt to the diminished amount of their chemical messenger. Then when dopamine becomes available again in normal amounts (when the patient starts taking levodopa), these cells respond in an exaggerated manner. It seems probable also that other nerve cells which do not normally process levodopa can assume this function. They can convert it to dopamine, but they may release it inappropriately at the wrong times in response to the wrong signals and deliver it to unusual places. These adaptations do not seem to be reversed when levodopa therapy is begun. The involuntary movements do not diminish with time on continued treatment. No tolerance to this side effect appears to develop.

MENTAL EFFECTS OF LEVODOPA

Many patients describe a feeling of being more alert after first starting levodopa treatment. They appear more attentive and more spontaneous in their activity. They become more talkative, and they seem to have more initiative and to take more interest in the world around them. Some also complain of a feeling of nervousness, of an inner restlessness, or even "jitteriness." They may also have trouble sleeping at night. These effects are somewhat reminiscent of the effects of amphetamine and related drugs often given to combat drowsiness. This is not surprising because amphetamine works in the brain by activating the normal dopamine cells. Essentially, amphetamine causes these cells to release more dopamine than they normally would in the course of their usual traffic with other nerve cells. The actions of amphetamine can be blocked by drugs which block the action of dopamine. Usually the nervousness, restlessness, and insomnia subside after a few weeks of continuing treatment. If necessary, they can be controlled with minor tranquilizing drugs.

Another similar activating effect experienced by occasional patients is vivid dreaming. They may not have dreamed in years, but after starting levodopa treatment they again enjoy dreaming. Usually this is pleasant, but excessively vivid dreams may be distressing; rarely, they amount to nightmares. The simplest way of dealing with this problem is to avoid taking a bedtime dose of levodopa or to make the bedtime dose somewhat smaller. This effect also tends to diminish in time on continued treatment.

It is often difficult to tell whether a change in behavior after levodopa treatment is begun is an improvement or a side effect. The patient who finds he or she has more energy and can resume doing many things around the house that had been turned over to others is improved. However, the spouse and family may complain that the patient is too "bossy," "stubborn," or "demanding." In some cases it seems to me that the family resents the patient reasserting a former dominance, whereas at other times it is clear that a personality change has indeed occurred.

Increased sexual interest and activity has been described as a side effect. The increased interest is evident in a number of patients. In most, it has been a partial recovery toward normal, although in some cases the increased sexual activity seemed excessive and inappropriate. Most patients, however, experience no change in libido. Some years ago the alleged effect of levodopa on sexual life attracted the interest of the press. Many of my patients who read the news-paper reports humorously asked me what I had left out of their pills! Because of these reports, levodopa has been tried in the treatment of impotence, but it has proved ineffective.

Rarely, levodopa seems to induce a hyperactive behavior in which the affected patient becomes agitated or "nervous," attempts too many projects, writes numerous letters, calls everyone he knows on the telephone, and plans ambitious undertakings. This behavior may occur episodically. I have known several patients who did foolish, unusual things during these episodes. One man bought a red sports car he could not drive.

Rarely, also, levodopa can provoke episodes of confused, irra-tional behavior. These may include visual halluciations similar to those the anticholinergic drugs can produce. However, levodopa is much less prone to produce such effects than any of the other anti-Parkinson drugs. Patients who are especially sensitive to the hal-lucinogenic effect of these drugs should avoid all drugs, including sleep medications, antihistamines, cough suppressants, etc., except levodopa. Even then the levodopa dosage should be adjusted very cautiously.

Levadopa can provoke a nervous breakdown in certain susceptible persons, primarily those who have had nervous breakdowns in the past or who are latent or inactive schizophrenics. Levadopa can reactivate latent schizophrenia into a full-blown psychosis. It can also exacerbate ongoing schizophrenia. This is really not surprising if we recall that the major tranquilizers so useful in treating schiz-ophrenia block dopamine in the brain. Indeed, some believe that schizophrenia is a disorder of brain dopamine due to overproduction of dopamine or to an abnormal sensitivity of certain regions of the brain to dopamine.

An increase in the dosage in an attempt to gain better control of the symptoms may initiate a train of mental symptoms in patients who have been on long-term treatment. Vivid dreams and night-mares lead to insomnia. Sleep medications prove to be of little help and insomnia persists. Agitation and confusion occur during the day, followed by visual hallucinations, which are often dream-like in quality. This situation has been aptly termed the "dopa madness." To reverse it requires reducing the dosage of levodopa. In severe cases, hospitalization for a drug holiday may be needed.

Depression or melancholia is not uncommon among parkinsonian patients. Some physicians have reported that levodopa may exacerbate or provoke depression. Others have thought it might help alleviate depression; most feel it has no effect. In my own experience, either effect may occur. Depression may be masked by the symptoms of parkinsonism so that when the latter are relieved by levodopa treatment the depression then becomes apparent. Therefore one should be alert to the possibility of depression. Effective treatment for depression is available and may be used in combination with levodopa therapy. Levodopa need not normally be discontinued. Usually both conditions can be treated simultaneously. The drugs commonly used to treat depression—the "tricyclics," such as imipramine (Tofranil) and amitriptyline (Elavil)—may readily be used at the same time as levodopa and may even work better with levodopa than if used alone.

There is, however, one group of drugs sometimes used to treat depression that should *never* under any circumstances be given to a patient on levodopa therapy. This is the group of *monoamine oxidase inhibitor* drugs. By blocking the action of the enzyme *monoamine oxidase* these drugs turn off the body's normal mechanism for preventing excessive accumulation of dopamine, adrenaline and noradrenaline. Levodopa can be metabolized to all three of these substances, and so they accumulate in abnormal amounts in the body very rapidly if levodopa and a monoamine oxidase inhibitor drug are taken together. The results are similar to the effects of an overdose of adrenaline. The heart pounds rapidly, the blood pressure shoots up very high, and palpitations, shortness of breath, nausea, vomiting, severe headaches, agitation, convulsions, and coma may result. There is a serious possibility of provoking a heart attack or a cerebral hemorrhage. Similar reactions can occur when a monoamine oxidase inhibitor is combined with a variety of other drugs, such as amphetamine, and even with certain foods, especially cheddar cheese and certain wines. In fact, since this reaction was first

noted in patients who ate cheese while on treatment with a monoamine oxidase inhibitor, it has been called the "cheese reaction."
The monoamine oxidase inhibitor drugs in current use include the
following: pargyline (Eutonyl), phenelzine (Nardil), and tranylcypromine (Parnate).

LOW BLOOD PRESSURE

Levodopa also accumulates in other parts of the nervous system.
It is believed to enter sympathetic nerves, which control the heart
and blood vessels throughout the body. In these nerves, levodopa
simply enters the normal metabolic pathway for the formation of
adrenaline and noradrenaline. However, because it is present in
unnatural amounts, it may interfere with the normal function of the
sympathetic nervous system. The result may be episodes of rapid
heart beat (rapid pulse), which may be felt as palpitations. Elevation
or depression of blood pressure may also occur. Indeed, dopamine
is now employed as a drug in its own right to treat low blood
pressure; it is injected by vein to raise blood pressure as an emergency measure in patients with very low blood pressure following
serious injuries or major surgery, a condition known as "shock."
However, in patients on levodopa treatment, the blood pressure
usually tends to decrease. In fact, in some patients it may fall to
such low levels that symptoms such as faintness, dizziness, and
lightheadedness result. Levodopa by mouth very rarely causes brief
periods of high blood pressure. Low blood pressure is by far the
most common of the side effects involving the circulatory system.
A striking feature is that the blood pressure may be normal if measured in the lying or sitting position, only to fall when the patient
stands up. This occurs because the blood pools in the legs. Normally
the sympathetic nervous system acts on the blood vessels to counter
the effects of gravity and maintain a uniform flow of blood to the
head. This is accomplished by constriction of blood vessels in the
legs, which prevents accumulation of blood in the leg muscles. The
sympathetic nervous system is somewhat impaired in some patients
with Parkinson's disease. The effect of levodopa on these nerves

may further impair their function so that they may not be able to prevent the pooling of blood in the legs when the patient stands up.

This side effect of levodopa may be countered by several measures. A simple, frequently effective one is to administer salt tablets. Several tablets a day (containing 0.25 or 0.5 grams of sodium chloride) suffice for most patients having this side effect. Another measure is to wear elastic stockings to prevent the pooling of blood in the veins. This is especially useful in patients with varicose veins, which may pool a considerable volume of blood. A variety of such stockings are available, some readymade, others made to order. The latter are more expensive but are also more effective and durable. They should be put on in the morning *before* getting out of bed.

If these countermeasures are not sufficient, the patient's physician may wish to try the drug fluorohydrocortisone. As the name implies, this drug is related to cortisone, the hormone of the adrenal cortex, which is used to treat severe arthritis and allergic reactions, among other conditions. Fluorohydrocortisone is a synthetic hormone that controls the metabolism of sodium chloride. It causes the kidney to retain more sodium chloride—and release less of it into the urine—than it would otherwise do. It is a very potent drug and has been helpful in the rare patient with severe low blood pressure complicating parkinsonism.

Because the action of the bladder is under the influence of the sympathetic nerves, some weakening of bladder function is very occasionally experienced by patients when they first start levodopa treatment. The effect is relatively mild, indeed much milder than the similar effect of the anticholinergic drugs. It is a relatively rare side effect of levodopa and seems to occur only in men. Rarely, patients report that they have more constipation on levodopa treatment, but I am not convinced that this is in fact a real effect of the drug.

DISCOLORATION OF URINE AND SWEAT

A major portion of the levodopa absorbed by the intestine is removed from the circulation by the kidneys. The kidneys rapidly convert it to dopamine and then to a series of inactive substances. Some of these are pigments called melanins. They range in color from orange to red to brown and finally to black. The pigments are more likely to be formed if the urine is alkaline. Drops of urine reacting with alkaline materials, such as dried bleach in underclothing or bedsheets, may produce reddish or brownish stains. Many patients have been frightened by such stains, mistaking them for blood. Occasionally patients note after passing urine that the water in the toilet bowl is tinged with red. This is especially likely to occur if the bowl was recently treated with some disinfectant solution. In case of doubt, it is best of course to consult a physician. The urine can very quickly be examined to ascertain whether there has been bleeding into the urinary tract.

A very small amount of levodopa may also be secreted by the sweat glands. Rarely, some dark beads of sweat result and stain undergarments.

INTERACTIONS WITH OTHER DRUGS

Patients are often concerned if a drug prescribed by another doctor for some acute illness may interfere with their levodopa. For example, they may have been given an antibiotic to treat the flu or some other infection. Or perhaps a doctor has prescribed an antihistamine to control some hayfever symptoms, or the dentist may want to administer Novocain before drilling. Many other examples come to mind. In nearly all of these situations, there is no problem. Levodopa is a particularly forgiving drug and can be used with almost anything. Only a few interactions of any significance have been encountered.

The number one "no-no" is to combine a monoamine oxidase inhibitor drug with levodopa. I have already explained the potentially dangerous interactions that can occur when levodopa and a monoamine oxidase inhibitor are taken together. Under no circumstances should these agents be combined.

Monoamine oxidase inhibiting drugs had been tried in the treatment of parkinsonism before the introduction of levodopa, but were soon abandoned as ineffective. They were tried again in combination with levodopa in the early days of experimentation with levodopa. The idea was to enhance and prolong the effect of levodopa. Although these drugs did enhance the effect of a given dose of levodopa, they did not prolong the duration of the response and, unfortunately, they produced episodes of high blood pressure and very rapid pulse rates. My own experience with these drugs convinced me that even in small doses they were dangerous and unpredictable. In any case, the same benefits could be obtained by merely increasing the dose of levodopa.

Recently, some patients have been treated with small doses of tranylcypromine (Parnate). The evidence that doing this is truly helpful and without risk is inconclusive and I do not advise it.

Aside from this one serious interaction, there is little to fear. All that can happen is that the effect of levodopa may be diminished. The major tranquilizer drugs, which act by blocking the action of dopamine in the nervous system, simply diminish the actions of levodopa. Therefore they should not be taken by patients on levodopa therapy. Also, patients should be cautious about taking vitamin preparations containing large amounts of vitamin B_6 (pyridoxine) because this vitamin can antagonize the effects of levodopa. The mechanism of this somewhat surprising interaction is explained in Chapter 10. There is also some evidence that the drug papaverine, often prescribed in the hope of improving blood flow to the brain in elderly persons, may antagonize the action of levodopa. Since this drug is ineffective anyway, there is no reason Parkinson patients on levodopa treatment should take it.

There is no problem in giving antibiotics, analgesics, antihistamines, vaccines, "flu shots," or Novocain anesthesia to Parkinson patients on levodopa treatment.

ENZYME INHIBITOR DRUGS

The conversion of L-DOPA to dopamine as described on page 83 is controlled by a specific enzyme bearing the impressive scientific name L-aromatic amino acid decarboxylase. When we speak of levodopa metabolism, we commonly refer to this enzyme by the short name, DOPA decarboxylase. A number of drugs inhibit this enzyme. They are therefore known to the pharmacologist as DOPA decarboxylase inhibitors. Several of these inhibitors greatly increase the effect of a given dose of levodopa in Parkinson patients, and two of them are used in combination with levodopa: carbidopa and bensarizide. The combination of carbidopa and levodopa is marketed under the trade name Sinemet in a single tablet containing both drugs. A similar combination containing levodopa and bensarizide is marketed under the name Madopar, but this is not available in the United States. Each of these formulations is available in several strengths, as shown in the Appendix. In my experience, these two preparations are very similar in their effect.

These drugs modify the body's metabolism of levodopa by inhibiting the enzyme DOPA decarboxylase and thus preventing the conversion of levodopa to dopamine. The key to their value in treating parkinsonism is that they are unable to enter the brain. The brain differs from all other organs in having the ability to regulate the admission of substances traveling through the body in the circulation. It has in effect, a highly selective barrier. We call it the blood-brain barrier. It admits levodopa but not dopamine. Similarly, it does not admit carbidopa or bensarizide. As a result of this curious circumstance, carbidopa and bensarizide inhibit the conversion of levodopa to dopamine throughout the body *except* in the brain. Consequently, these greatly increase the proportion of levodopa taken by mouth that ultimately reaches the brain and is converted to dopamine. In effect, they protect the levodopa until it has a chance to reach the brain. The protection is not complete, but it is quite significant. In practice, approximately 80% less levodopa need be taken by mouth when the combination treatment is used than when levodopa is used alone. This means that a patient who needs 5 grams of levodopa to control his symptoms now needs only 1 gram. Instead of ten 0.5-gram tablets of levodopa a day, he needs only four tablets of Sinemet or Madopar containing 0.25 grams of levodopa each. Taking four small pills instead of ten large ones is a matter of some convenience. However, the major bonus of combining levodopa with a decarboxylase inhibitor is that it largely abolishes the action of levodopa on the vomiting center. The reason for this is that this area does not hide behind the blood-brain barrier. To do its work, the vomiting center must be able to sample the various substances traveling in the circulation. Thus carbidopa and bensarizide gain access to the vomiting center and prevent the formation of dopamine there. The practical consequences are considerable. First, a patient just starting levodopa therapy need not begin with very small doses and build up slowly over a period of months to the full dosage while waiting for the vomiting center to develop tolerance for levodopa. Instead, the patient can reach full dosage within a matter of days. Second, the various precautions discussed above to minimize levodopa-induced nausea and vomiting can now usually be ignored. Thus dose schedules can be set up without regard to mealtimes but only in accord with the patient's need. The patient who requires levodopa immediately upon arising in the morning need not wait until after breakfast but can take the combination tablet even before getting out of bed. The patient who needs levodopa every 2 or 3 hours to maintain a smooth response throughout the day need no longer wait until the next meal but can take the combination tablet on an empty stomach. For these reasons, treatment with Sinemet and Madopar is much more convenient and agreeable to both patient and physician. Levodopa is now rarely used alone.

It must be admitted, of course, that all is not perfect even in the most perfect of all possible worlds. There are a very few patients who still feel some nausea despite taking levodopa in combination with carbidopa or bensarizide. These few patients must heed the precautions discussed above and which were learned in the early days of levodopa therapy. One reason for the failure of the inhibitor to protect all patients completely from activation of the vomiting center is that the amount of carbidopa in the smaller tablet, the 10/100 tablet—containing 10 milligrams of carbidopa and 100 milligrams (or 0.10 grams) of levodopa—may not be sufficient to prevent the formation of some dopamine in the vomiting center. The obvious solution to this is to take an additional amount of carbidopa separately. This is provided in the 25/100 tablet containing 25 mg of carbidopa. With this yellow, scored tablet, it is possible to use a half tablet, that is, 12½/50 mg, and still have enough carbidopa to prevent nausea. Since the introduction of the 25/100 tablet, nausea has been a rare occurrence. Those rare patients still having nausea may be helped by using diphenidol (Vontrol) or trimethobenzamide (Tigan).

Patients who are doing well on levodopa alone need not change to the combined preparations. Although many physicians feel that patients do slightly better on the combined treatment than on levodopa alone in an equivalent dosage, all other things being equal, some patients are unable to see any difference between the two treatment regimens. In fact, there are a few patients who seem to fare better on levodopa alone. The reason is that it is more difficult to make small adjustments in dosage with the levodopa-decarboxylase inhibitor combination. The difference between a half tablet and a full tablet represents a much greater increment in the amount of levodopa delivered to the brain than a comparable change in dosage of levodopa tablets. Also, the more efficient delivery of levodopa to the brain results not only in a stronger therapeutic effect but also in a greater severity of those side effects that are due to the action of levodopa in the brain. Thus patients who are very sensitive to the actions of levodopa and require only small doses may respond better to levodopa alone than to the combination.

CHAPTER 8

Imitators of Dopamine

No one who can remember what parkinsonism was like before levodopa can doubt that it was a very great improvement over the drug treatments previously available. Great as this improvement was, however, levodopa was clearly not the final answer. From the earliest days of levodopa treatment, physicians have yearned for a still more effective drug. They have thought that some of the limitations of levodopa treatment stem from the fact that it has no effect itself but must first be converted to dopamine. For a number of theoretical reasons it has seemed desirable to find a substance that would not need to be converted to the active agent but could act the same way as dopamine. It is hoped, then, that some of the side effects of levodopa might not occur.

Many drugs directly imitating the action of dopamine have been tested in Parkinson patients. At least one of the drugs, bromocriptine, is now regularly used in the treatment of parkinsonism. More are in various stages of development, and it seems likely that some of these agents will have considerable importance in the years ahead. These "imitators" of dopamine are properly termed, in the language of the pharmacologist, *dopamine receptor agonists*. To understand the meaning of this term it is necessary to think for a moment about how dopamine works in the nervous system.

I have described dopamine as a chemical messenger essential to the normal function of the brain. It is the means whereby the nerve cells of the substantia nigra communicate with the corpus striatum.

105

These nerve cells form and store dopamine; they release it in the corpus striatum. The nerve cells of the striatum receive this messenger at special receptor sites on their surfaces, which recognize and respond to dopamine, but not to other naturally occurring chemical messengers. For example, the dopamine receptors will pay little attention to epinephrine, norepinephrine, serotonin, or other chemical messengers that are also normally present in the corpus striatum. They are highly specific for dopamine and thus we may think of them as *dopamine receptors*.

Although the dopamine receptors are very selective regarding which chemical messengers they will recognize, they can be fooled. Many substances are now known to act at the dopamine receptors in much the same way dopamine does. Drugs that can activate a receptor are known collectively as *agonists* of that receptor, in contrast to those drugs which can block the receptor, and are thus termed *antagonists*.

The first dopamine receptor agonist to be tested in Parkinson patients was apomorphine. This drug has long been useful in medical practice as an emetic. It activates the dopamine receptors in the vomiting center and is used to induce vomiting. The late Dr. George Cotzias hypothesized that it might also act on the dopamine receptors in the corpus striatum and thereby control the symptoms of parkinsonism. In fact, it had earlier been reported by Dr. Albert Schwab in Boston in the 1950s that an injection of apomorphine temporarily reduced the tremor of Parkinson's disease. Dr. Cotzias gave apomorphine by mouth to a small number of patients in much the same way he had prescribed levodopa. That is, he started treatment with small doses which he gradually increased to allow his patients time to develop tolerance to the emetic action of apomorphine. With care and persistence he was able to reach substantial doses and these did in fact yield significant relief of the symptoms of parkinsonism. He estimated that apomorphine was 40 to 50% as effective as levodopa. However, the blood tests he carried out in his patients indicated that there was a toxic effect on the kidneys. High doses of apomorphine could not be be used as a sustained treatment. Cotzias and his colleagues searched for other drugs which might have the same properties. They tested a synthetic agent similar to apomorphine, N-methyl aporphine. The results were similar. Again there was evidence of a toxic effect on the kidneys.

Although this work failed to produce a new treatment, it did show that a dopamine receptor agonist could have a significant anti-Parkinson effect, and gave impetus to the search for better and less toxic agonists. A totally different drug, piribedil (Trivastal) was also found, somewhat unexpectedly, to be a dopamine receptor agonist. It too was tested in Parkinson patients but was abandoned as relatively ineffective. Then, a synthetic analogue of ergotamine, the alkaloid drug used in treating migraine, was found to be a powerful dopamine receptor agonist. This new drug, bromocriptine (Parlodel) appeared to have some advantages over levodopa in animal experiments. For example, its action lasted for 5 to 6 hr, whereas levodopa acted for only 2 to 3 hr in the same animals. It was also much more potent. A very small dose seemed equal in effect to a very large dose of levodopa.

Bromocriptine was initially tried in Parkinson patients by Dr. Donald Calne and his colleagues in London, England in 1973. Definite effects were found with modest doses. These results were soon confirmed by other investigators. After a decade of extensive experimental treatment at various doses, alone, and in combination with other drugs, the role of bromocriptine in the treatment of parkinsonism is well established.

It is about 50% as effective as levodopa in relieving the symptoms of parkinsonism. Although it can be used alone in some patients for a period of time, it is most useful when used in combination with levodopa. Unfortunately, it cannot fully substitute for levodopa. Probably, the most important useful quality of this drug is that its action lasts longer than that of levodopa. It is thus most helpful in patients with the "on-off" effect who enjoy only a short-duration response from each dose of levodopa, even when taking it every 2 to 3 hr. Bromocriptine can reduce the fluctuations, making the "on" phases last longer and the "off" phases shorter and milder. I have found it especially useful for patients suffering painful muscle cramps in their "off" phases.

The side effects are similar to those of levodopa. Loss of appetite, nausea, vomiting, lowering of blood pressure, involuntary movements, agitation, vivid dreams, nightmares, confusion, and hallucinations have all been observed. Tolerance to the nausea and vomiting takes place rapidly. Usually, only mild nausea is encountered, and subsides within a matter of days. Loss of appetite also disappears quickly and may be replaced after a period of time by an increase in appetite. A few of my patients have complained of gaining weight but this has been minimal. Rarely, blood pressure has fallen sufficiently to cause light-headedness, dizziness, and faintness. Rarely, also, bromocriptine seems to activate long quiescent peptic ulcer disease.

The major and most troublesome side effects have been mental disturbances. In the mildest cases, the patient displays an unusual suspiciousness of loved ones and friends. This may be followed by anxiety, insomnia, and vivid dreams. If the drug is continued, episodes of confusion and visual hallucinations may develop. In the severest cases, the patient is irrational and agitated. The propensity of bromocriptine to induce these toxic mental effects is much greater than that of levodopa or the anticholinergic drugs. Of course, as with similar side effects with other drugs, these undesired manifestations subside rapidly after the drug is stopped.

Despite its side effects and limitations, bromocriptine is a useful addition to the list of drugs now available to treat parkinsonism. It is not for every patient and it serves mainly as a supplement to levodopa. Used cautiously in specific situations, it can be very helpful. Unfortunately, it is available only in a 2.5 and 5 mg tablet marketed under the name "parlodel." It is a very complex molecule and very difficult to synthesize. Consequently, its cost is considerable. Although some benefit may be seen with very low doses of 2.5 to 5 mg three times daily, to obtain a significant effect requires much larger doses of 10 to 20 mg three times daily or even more. The high cost of the drug makes it impractical to maintain treatment at such doses for most patients. As a result, many patients who might benefit from treatment with a dopamine receptor agonist are not presently receiving such treatment. Perhaps the major contribution of bromocriptine is that it firmly established the potential of the dopamine receptor agonists as anti-Parkinson drugs, and stimulated research on the dopamine receptor and the development of many similar drugs.

Several other dopamine receptor agonists have been tried in Parkinson patients, notably lergotrile, lisuride, and pergolide. Lergotrile has been abandoned because of toxic effects on the liver. Lisuride and pergolide remain experimental drugs at this time. Experience with these drugs has been limited. Their clinical effects seem to be very similar to those of bromocriptine. They are more potent and may produce less mental side effects, but it is still too early to say precisely what place they will ultimately have in the treatment of parkinsonism. Unfortunately, clinical work with pergolide was delayed in the United States because of a report suggesting that it may cause skipped heart beats and other irregularities of the heart rate. The Federal Food and Drug Administration placed a moratorium on pergolide in August 1981. Clinical investigators working with the drug were prohibited from enrolling additional patients in their trials but could continue treatment in patients already receiving the drug. Several hundred patients have now been on pergolide treatment, some for over 3 years. The accumulating experience indicates that it will be a useful agent especially in treating patients with the "on-off" effect. It should not be expected to replace levodopa; rather, it will work best when used in combination with levodopa as has been the case with bromocriptine.

None of the dopamine receptor agonists presently available or under clinical trial is sufficiently effective to warrant being used as the initial nor as the only drug in the treatment of parkinsonism. None quite equals the action of levodopa. The reason for this difference is still not clear. Experiments in animal models of parkinsonism suggest that some effect of levodopa other than the replenishment of brain dopamine stores may be important. I emphasized in Chapter 1 the depletion of dopamine in parkinsonism. There is also, however, a depletion of norepinehprine stores. Levodopa treatment may also, at least partially, correct the norepinephrine deficiency. The dopamine receptor agonists do not activate the brain norepinephrine receptors.

Another explanation for the limited effects of the dopamine receptor agonists studied to date may lie in the recent discovery that there are at least two major types of dopamine receptors. These have been designated the D-1 and D-2 receptors on the basis of certain distinct chemical properties. Dopamine activates both receptors. Bromocriptine activates only the D-2 receptor; it is actually an ANTAgonist of the D-1 receptor! Pergolide is a weak D-1 and strong D-2 agonist. Only one selective D-1 agonist is presently known but it is not yet available for human use. Studies carried out by Doctors Gershanik and Heikkila, and myself at Rutgers Medical School indicate that the two receptors have different functions, and that normal bodily movement requires activation of both types of receptors. Thus, the further development of drugs capable of acting selectively and exclusively at only one or the other of these dopamine receptors may make possible a more effective anti-Parkinson treatment.

CHAPTER 9

Special Remedies for Special Symptoms

In the preceding chapter I described the major anti-Parkinson drugs: the anticholinergics, levodopa, the dopamine receptor agonists, and amantadine. These drugs act on the parkinsonian state as a whole and are not directed specifically against any one symptom. In general, they relieve all or at least most symptoms related to the classic triad: tremor, rigidity, and bradykinesia. There remains a miscellaneous group of drugs whose acquaintance many patients are apt to make sooner or later. They are not specific for parkinsonian symptoms but rather are used to treat symptoms which are very common, such as insomnia, anxiety, constipation, etc. Some discussion of these drugs seems appropriate because Parkinson patients may react differently to these commonly used agents, and some of these drugs may interact adversely with the major anti-Parkinson drugs.

PROPRANOLOL

The drug propranolol (Inderal) is used mainly to treat irregularity of the pulse and, to a lesser extent, to control high blood pressure. It may be used for these purposes in Parkinson patients with heart disease, irregular heart rate, or high blood pressure. It may also be used to protect the heart from the possibility of levodopa causing palpitations or episodes of abnormal heart rhythm in patients who are subject to palpitations.

Propranolol, however, has also been used occasionally because it seems to have a favorable effect on tremor, at least in some patients. Because the drug has an important action on the heart, it must be used with care. It is not recommended for asthmatics or in patients who have had heart failure since it may exacerbate these conditions.

A very occasional patient who still has some disturbing tremor despite good effects on other symptoms of Parkinson's disease may enjoy a good response to this drug. Unfortunately, propranolol has no effect on other symptoms.

Propranolol is commonly used today to treat the symptom of tremor in the condition known as "benign essential tremor" or "familial tremor." This is sometimes confused with parkinsonism because the tremor often bears a superficial resemblance. Persons with essential or familial tremor do not develop any of the other manifestations of Parkinson's disease, however, even after 40 to 50 years. On closer examination, their tremor differs in a number of respects from that of Parkinson's disease. One of these differences is that the tremor commonly involves the head and the voice; this rarely if ever occurs in Parkinson's disease. Another feature is that essential tremor usually runs in families; in nearly all instances, one parent also had the condition. Finally, essential tremor responds differently to various drugs. In particular, it can be suppressed for a few hours by alcohol. The tremor of Parkinson's disease is not reduced by alcohol. A highball or a glass of sherry dramatically diminishes the former for a few hours but not the latter. The various minor tranquilizers may also effectively reduce essential tremor, paralleling the action of alcohol. Levodopa has no effect on essential tremor but, as we noted, can greatly reduce or abolish the tremor of Parkinson's disease.

Several new drugs, closely related to propranolol, have recently been released. One of these, metoprolol (Lopressor), is used primarily in treating high blood pressure. It is not as effective as propranolol against tremor, but has much less risk of exacerbating asthma.

MINOR TRANQUILIZERS AND HYPNOTICS

Minor tranquilizers are sometimes prescribed for patients with tremor persisting despite treatment with the usual anti-Parkinson drugs and to relieve the sense of inner restlessness and nervousness which may occur as a symptom of Parkinson's disease or as a side effect of the anti-Parkinson drugs. Those most commonly used are chlordiazepoxide (Librium), diazepam (Valium), oxazepam (Serax), and meprobamate (Equanil and Miltown). These drugs are called minor tranquilizers to distinguish them from the major tranquilizers, such as chlorpromazine (Thorazine), trifluoperazine (Stelazine), and haloperidol (Haldol), which are used primarily in psychiatric practice to treat severe mental illness. The major tranquilizers, as we noted earlier, block the action of dopamine in the brain and consequently can cause parkinsonism. They therefore should not normally be given to Parkinson patients. The minor tranquilizers are entirely different and do not cause parkinsonism. They may, in fact, be quite useful but should be used sparingly and only as needed.

The minor tranquilizers can cause drowsiness, incoordination, dizziness, and confusion, and occasionally seem to increase the bradykinesia or slowness of movement of Parkinson's disease. Moreover, some persons may become psychologically dependent on or habituated to these drugs. Patients who use these drugs heavily for a period of time and then suddenly stop taking them may suffer withdrawal symptoms, including nervousness, agitation, and even (rarely) convulsions. However, I have never encountered a Parkinson patient who became dependent on these drugs, perhaps because I am careful to prescribe them sparingly.

Phenobarbital has also been used as a minor tranquilizer for many years as well as a drug to induce sleep at night. Parkinson patients should avoid phenobarbital and other barbiturates for the same reason they should use the other minor tranquilizers sparingly. The barbiturates may aggravate the bradykinesia of parkinsonism and can also be habit-forming.

What then can the Parkinson patient with insomnia take to induce sleep? Preferably, of course, nothing. If levodopa (whether used alone or as Sinemet) seems to be responsible for insomnia, the bedtime dose should be avoided; if the drug is necessary, it might be reduced 50%. Several old nonmedical tricks may be quite helpful in inducing sleep at night, including a warm drink (such as a glass of warm milk) or even a brandy at bedtime. If insomnia is still a problem, a mild sedative such as chloral hydrate may be used. This is a very old and mild short-acting sedative that leaves no hangover and is least apt of all the available hypnotics to cause confusion. It is made in the form of 0.25- and 0.5-gram capsules. Your physician may direct you to take one capsule on retiring and if necessary to take another capsule an hour later. Two capsules (1.0 gram) may be used on retiring if one is not effective.

The drug flurazepam (Dalmane) is a commonly prescribed hypnotic introduced a few years ago. It is closely related to diazepam (Valium) and may also increase the bradykinesia of parkinsonism. Thus I generally avoid this drug in treating my patients.

The drug glutethimide (Doriden) is commonly prescribed to help patients sleep at night. Because it tends to drop the blood pressure, especially in elderly subjects, it is used cautiously. However, it does have some anticholinergic properties and thus may provide some small degree of anti-Parkinson activity. Moreover, unlike the barbiturates, it does not exacerbate the bradykinesia of parkinsonism. Thus it is useful in occasional Parkinson patients who need something stronger than chloral hydrate. Glutethimide is available in two sizes: 0.25- and 0.5-gram white scored tablets which can easily be divided in half if necessary. Usually the smaller-dose tablet is sufficient. In patients with low blood pressure and in those prone to developing vivid dreaming, nightmares, mental confusion, or hallucinations on anticholinergic drugs, it should be used very carefully if at all.

OVER-THE-COUNTER SEDATIVES

Parkinson patients should avoid over-the-counter sedatives such as Compoz, Sominex, Sleep-eze, Nytol, and others. These preparations all contain scopolamine (hyoscine) in quantities comparable to those formerly employed in treating parkinsonism (see comments on solanaceous alkaloids in Chapter 6) as one of the active ingredients. They also contain an over-the-counter antihistamine, methapyrilene hydrochloride, which like other antihistamines also has some anticholinergic activity. The addition of these agents to a Parkinson patient's existing drug regimen, which may already include some anticholinergic agents, may carry the patient over the threshold of anticholinergic toxicity. Consequently Parkinson patients are less able to tolerate the side effects commonly produced by these medications. On the other hand, the anticholinergic properties of these formulations may have some beneficial effect on the symptoms of parkinsonism. Patients should consult their doctors before trying them, however, to minimize the chance of an unpleasant interaction with their own anti-Parkinson drug treatment.

DIURETICS

Swelling of the feet due to the accumulation of water in the tissues (edema) of the legs and feet is a common manifestation of parkinsonism. It is often more marked in one leg, nearly always the leg on the side where the first symptoms occurred. The causes of this swelling are not fully understood. One reason may be that there is less muscular activity in that limb due to the bradykinesia of parkinsonism. In any event, the swelling can be relieved by diuretic agents (that is, drugs which increase the volume of urine passed in a day). The milder common diuretic chlorothiazide (Diuril) and its derivative hydrochlorothiazide (Hydrodiuril) may effectively relieve this swelling. Usually only one dose once or twice a week is necessary. The drug should be taken only with a doctor's prescription.

If the swelling was induced by the drug amantadine (Symmetrel), it should subside when that drug is stopped although it may require several weeks to disappear. If varicose veins are present, elastic hose may be helpful. Further treatment may be advised by the doctor.

LAXATIVES

Chronic constipation is a familiar symptom of Parkinson's disease. It results from a general slowing of the muscular action of the bowel or of muscular action in other organs. As mentioned earlier, constipation is also often exacerbated by the drugs used in treating parkinsonism. The tendency of Parkinson patients to drink little water is a further complicating factor. Consequently many patients need to take laxatives.

I urge patients to try natural means of maintaining normal bowel habits. This means making an effort to drink more water, to eat adequate roughage and high-fiber foods, and to ingest prunes, prune juice, or figs regularly. Failing all this, one must resort to laxatives. Several classes of laxatives need be considered.

First, there are bulk laxatives which work by retaining water in the stools. Patients who pass small, hard stools—really dehydrated stools—may benefit from this measure alone. A common laxative in this class is Metamucil, available over the counter. A tablespoonful stirred in one glass of water a day may suffice.

Another useful preparation is the fecal softener dioctyl sodium sulfosuccinate. A great many proprietary over-the-counter preparations containing this ingredient are available. One capsule one, two, or three times daily may be used. Generally, these are used on a regular daily maintenance basis by Parkinson patients.

If these measures are inadequate, the "irritant" laxatives which stimulate the bowel directly may be required. Milder ones such as bisacodyl (Dulcolax) are preferable. Some preparations combine such a stimulant with the fecal softeners mentioned above. The pharmacist can give advice about a suitable one, or the patient can check the label on the packages on the supermarket shelf, looking for the two ingredients dioctyl sodium sulfosuccinate and bisacodyl.

Finally, many patients have a laxative habit acquired long before Parkinson's disease developed. They may prefer to continue using their old favorites. As a last resort, enemas may be required to maintain adequate evacuation.

ARTIFICIAL TEARS

The reduced frequency of spontaneous eye blink which is common in parkinsonism may result in some redness and dryness of the eyes and eyelids. The lids may become encrusted. Patients feel some irritation, a dry, burning feeling in the eyes. Usually the major anti-Parkinson drugs restore eye blink to more normal frequency; with improvement in the normal "windshield wiper" function of the eyelids, these symptoms are relieved. However, if there is still some eye discomfort, irrigating the eyes with artificial tear solutions may be helpful. Various preparations of artificial tears can be purchased at local drug stores over the counter. They reproduce the salt concentration of natural tears. If symptoms are not relieved by this simple measure, medical advice should be sought.

TREATMENT FOR SEBORRHEA

The increased activity of the sebaceous gland of the skin in parkinsonism commonly results in a somewhat greasy appearance of the face and forehead (seborrhea) and occasionally in some irritation and inflammation of the skin (seborrheic dermatitis). The seborrhea and the secondary dermatitis are reduced by treatment, especially by levodopa, and are rarely serious problems. Seborrhea can be controlled by washing daily with bland or neutral soaps. A commonly used soap formulation is the acne aid bar available at most drug stores. Dermatitis responds to a variety of lotions containing small amounts of hydrocortisone or related agents, but these require a doctor's prescription.

A variety of hair lotions are available over the counter that may satisfactorily control excessive dandruff. One of the more effective contains selenium and is marketed under the name Selsun. A more concentrated solution of selenium is also available with a doctor's prescription. Many authorities advise that selenium preparations be used sparingly because they may cause hair loss if used excessively. It would be preferable to reserve them for a last resort and then use them only occasionally.

DRUGS FOR LEG CRAMPS

The painful leg cramps which sometimes occur as a symptom of parkinsonism are usually so transitory that no medication seems necessary. In some patients it appears that with high doses of levodopa the cramps become more severe and that they may disappear altogether if the dose is lowered substantially. This may be counted among the paradoxical effects of levodopa. Most commonly the cramps are nocturnal and seem very similar to the common nocturnal cramp which many people, not just parkinsonians, experience especially after strenuous exercise. A traditional and reasonably effective remedy for nocturnal cramps is quinine sulfate taken at bedtime in a dose of 200 or 300 mg. Quinine prevents the cramp or at least diminishes its severity. It works very well for some patients but not so well for others. Other drugs that may help include an antihistamine such as diphenhydramine (Benadryl) 50 mg or orphenadrine citrate (Norflex) 100 mg, or a muscle relaxer such as diazepam (Valium) 5 mg at bedtime. The relatively new drug, lioresal (Baclofen), promoted for the treatment of spasticity, may be useful in controlling painful leg cramps in parkinsonism. The recommended dose is 10 mg three times daily. Double this amount, however, may be needed to yield substantial relief. Some individuals, however, have difficulty tolerating these doses of lioresal owing to nausea, dizziness, and drowsiness. You should follow your doctor's instructions carefully in using this drug. Vitamin E (alpha-tocopherol) has been recommended by some physicians to prevent nocturnal cramps, but it has not been effective in my patients.

CHAPTER 10

Surgical Treatment of Parkinsonism

There remains a relatively limited role for surgical treatment in parkinsonism today. Fifteen years ago, however, brain surgery for the relief of Parkinson symptoms was performed with some frequency. With the advent of levodopa, surgical treatment was largely abandoned, although brain surgery is still used in certain other disorders characterized by tremors or other involuntary movements for which there is still no effective drug treatment. Some physicians argue that there are still a few Parkinson patients for whom operative treatment may be helpful. These would be the few patients who cannot tolerate levodopa or who have severe tremor despite optimal drug treatment and who are in good general health. I have rarely recommended brain surgery for relief of Parkinson's disease since 1967, the year I began to treat patients with levodopa. The benefits of levodopa treatment are so remarkable in contrast to the effects achieved with our best previous medical treatment that there simply has been very little need of operative treatment. Those patients who do poorly on levodopa or who for some reason cannot tolerate it may be considered for brain surgery.

Why discuss the surgical treatment of parkinsonism at all? The possibility of brain surgery is still entertained at times. It was once an important treatment that received considerable publicity and was done fairly frequently up to 15 years ago. Many patients have had such surgery and may wish to know about the present status of the operations they underwent. Moreover, the story of the various surgical procedures is not without some interest. Indeed, it still seems remarkable that symptoms reflecting a disease of the brain could be alleviated by deliberately inflicting additional damage.

The first surgical efforts to alleviate parkinsonism were made during the 1930s. Various destructive operations were carried out in which some region of the cerebral cortex was removed or fibers deep in the brain were cut. The idea, stated somewhat crudely, was simply to damage the motor pathways enough to diminish tremor and rigidity without causing appreciable weakness. The results were mediocre and unpredictable, and the operations were relatively hazardous. Better procedures gradually evolved largely from thoughtful trial and error and astute observation of accidental results. Dr. Russell Myers, a neurosurgeon then working at the Long Island College Hospital in New York, made an interesting discovery in 1939 while operating on a Parkinson patient with a brain tumor. When he cut through a part of the corpus striatum, tremor and rigidity on the opposite side of the body suddenly diminished. Taking advantage of this chance observation, he repeated the procedure in several more Parkinson patients. After trying a number of modifications based on the knowledge of brain anatomy available at the time, he found that the best effect could be achieved by severing a very small bundle of nerve fibers, called the ansa lenticularis, rather deep in the brain. This bundle could be severed without producing any apparent ill effect, and the result was an appreciable reduction of tremor and rigidity in some cases. It was, however, very difficult to reach a small fiber bundle deep in the brain with a scalpel without inflicting damage to other brain structures. Complications were serious and frequent, and few operations were actually done.

Many surgeons around the world tried to solve the problem of cutting that small fiber bundle safely and effectively. The most successful procedure turned out to be a technique known as stereotactic surgery. The technique had long been employed in experimental brain surgery in animals. Drs. Henry T. Wycis and Ernest Spiegel, working at Temple University Hospital in Philadelphia, and Dr. Hiro Narabayashi working independently in Tokyo, adapted this technique to human patients in 1948. In this procedure a long needle is lowered into the brain through a small burr hole in the overlying skull. The direction and depth of the needle is carefully calculated from landmarks located on x-ray films of the patient's head. Placing the stereotactic needle in the desired place was a simple problem in spatial or three-dimensional geometry, and it could be done with considerable precision. When the needle was positioned satisfactorily, a solution of alcohol could be injected or an electrical current run from its tip, thereby destroying a small amount of brain tissue and severing the nerve fiber bundle. Drs. Wycis and Spiegel called their operation *"ansotomy."*

Various techniques of stereotactic surgery were developed. Perhaps the best known is the cryosurgery technique developed by Dr. Irving Cooper at St. Barnabas Hospital in New York. Dr. Cooper used a needle with a system of tiny tubes through which a refrigerant solution of liquid nitrogen could be pumped. The effect was literally to freeze a small area of brain. Prominent stereotaxic surgeons such as Dr. Mundinger in Germany, Dr. Leksell in Sweden, Dr. Siegfried in Switzerland, and Dr. Gillingham in Scotland used a radiofrequency current. With such refinements in technique, the stereotactic surgeons were able to limit the damage to a very small volume of brain tissue, of the order of several cubic millimeters. Various targets were selected by different surgeons, but they all involved the same nerve circuit; some surgeons caught it at its origin, some in the middle of its course, and others at its termination. Probably the best target proved to be the point of termination of that small fiber bundle Dr. Myers had identified back in 1939. That point is located in a region of the deep brain nucleus known as the thalamus. The stereotactic operation to destroy that part of the thalamus is thus termed *thalamotomy*.

Many thousands of patients were operated with these techniques at special centers throughout the world. Although these operations effectively reduced tremor and rigidity on one side of the body in most cases, they nevertheless stirred considerable controversy. No one could satisfactorily explain why the operations worked. Many thoughtful physicians were disturbed by the idea of treating a disease whose symptoms reflected some poorly understood brain dysfunction by injuring the brain and causing further change in function which was also poorly understood. Brain surgery could not cure or even alter the future progress of Parkinson's disease, and did not even relieve all the symptoms; it was mainly tremor and rigidity that were suppressed. Moreover, the operation had to be done twice, once for each side, if the symptoms on both sides of the body were to be relieved; and complications were much more frequent when both sides were operated.

The major risk of stereotactic brain surgery was the possibility that the needle, pushed blindly through the brain toward the desired target, might injure a blood vessel and cause bleeding or clotting. The result would be, in effect, a "stroke." There was also some difficulty because the standard measurements did not apply to all individuals, and as a result the needle might be placed a few millimeters off the target. Weakness of the arm or leg occasionally resulted, and in some the operation failed to give appreciable or lasting relief of tremor.

In the hands of experienced neurosurgeons, the results were generally quite good and the risks relatively small. The chance of dying as a result of the operation was less than 1%. There was a 2 to 3% chance of having some permanent weakness of the hand or leg on one side. Tremor and rigidity were markedly alleviated in 70 to 80% of cases. The results were not so good when the second side was operated. Especially troublesome was the development of slurring of speech and difficulty swallowing after the second operation. This occurred in as many as 15 to 20% of patients who were operated on twice.

To minimize risks, the surgeons were cautious in choosing which patients on whom to operate. Not surprisingly, the best results were obtained in young patients whose symptoms were mainly on one side and who were in good general health. Complications were more frequent in the elderly and especially in patients who had high blood pressure, diabetes, arteriosclerosis, heart disease, or other disorders affecting general health. It was also found that patients who had severe bradykinesia were not so likely to benefit from the operation as those who had only tremor and rigidity. Impairment of equilibrium on walking was not helped and sometimes was made worse. Speech dysfunction was not improved by surgery. Patients who were severely affected with Parkinson's disease were not likely to be improved.

As the neurosurgeons who specialized in this type of surgery gained experience, they narrowed their criteria for selecting patients for surgery. The criteria eventually became rather strict so that even the most aggressive and enthusiastic surgeons found only approximately 10% of Parkinson patients suitable for surgery. In the remaining 90% the risks of surgery were considered too great and the likelihood of real benefit too small. Thus to many patients and their doctors, stereotactic surgery, despite all the publicity it received, was rather disappointing.

There is no denying that stereotactic surgery did help many patients and that the results were occasionally dramatic. The operations were performed under local anesthesia with the patient awake throughout the procedure. Many patients described with wonderment and awe how they felt when the tremor suddenly stopped during the surgery. An excellent subjective account was given by the late Margaret Bourke White, the famous photographer. She wrote magazine articles and later a book about her experience of Parkinson's disease and her operation.

The publicity the operations received as a result of such individual accounts was a frequent cause of disappointment to the many patients who were not considered suitable for surgery. They had been led to hope for a miraculous cure by uncritical reports which appeared frequently in the popular press and in television documentaries. They sometimes had difficulty understanding why they too could not be helped. Many patients who were operated and enjoyed good relief of tremor and rigidity were also disappointed when, several years later, similar symptoms appeared in the opposite limbs. They had thought that the operation would cure the disease or at least prevent its further progression. The fact is, stereotactic surgery was nothing more than a symptomatic remedy for tremor and rigidity. It was not specific for Parkinson's disease but could alleviate these symptoms in many other conditions.

What we may call the surgical era in the treatment of parkinsonism came to an end when levodopa therapy was introduced during 1967–1970. Many stereotactic surgeons abandoned the operation altogether. A few continued mainly because they were using it for other purposes. In several neurosurgical centers Parkinson patients who still have some tremor despite levodopa treatment may be advised to have the operation. However, the number of patients who have been referred for such surgery and who are willing to undergo a brain operation has dwindled to a trickle.

There are still a few exceptional cases in which the operation seems justified. An example is a long-time patient of mine, Mrs. S. This pleasant lady, now in her mid-seventies, first came to see me 12 years ago with mild tremor of her left hand and foot. It did not interfere with her life or with her work as a cashier, and she did not wish to have brain surgery even though the drugs then available did not appreciably reduce the tremor. When it became available, I treated her with levodopa. The tremor disappeared only to be replaced by constant writhing involuntary movements of the left hand and foot, which Mrs. S. found just as disagreeable as the tremor. After trying various doses and schedules of levodopa, Mrs. S. finally decided to give up on levodopa and returned to her old medicines. The involuntary movements stopped, and the tremor recurred exactly as before the trial of levodopa. Today, 12 years after her tremor first appeared, she still has no symptom other than tremor of her left hand and foot. It has become slightly worse over the years and at times affects the chin, but there is no tremor on the right side and no other symptoms of Parkinson's disease. She retired at age 70 and has since been living a happy and very active life doing the many things she had dreamed of doing during the years she was working. She is still unwilling to have brain surgery even though chances are very good that her tremor could be abolished. She feels that her tremor does not bother her enough to warrant an operation on her brain.

Mrs. S. illustrates an important limitation of stereotactic surgery in the treatment of parkinsonism. The one symptom that this surgery can effectively relieve, regardless of its cause, is tremor, but patients who have only tremor and no other symptoms are rarely interested in having brain surgery. It is later in the course of Parkinson's disease, when slowness of movement, poor equilibrium, difficulty walking, and other, more disturbing symptoms appear that the patients are willing to undergo surgery. Unfortunately, these more-serious symptoms are not appreciably helped by stereotactic surgery and may even be made worse. Thus when the patients really need help, surgery is not effective. Mrs. S. represents the ideal candidate for surgery, but she simply will not have it. Although I believe that the operation would have benefited Mrs. S. had it been done when I first saw her, I cannot argue with her decision. It was hers to make, and she is still confident that she made the right choice.

CHAPTER 11

Dietary Considerations

Malnutrition can cause disturbances—even very serious disturbances—of the nervous system, including various paralyses, loss
of feeling, incoordination, convulsions, and mental deterioration;
but malnutrition has never caused parkinsonism. There is no known
nutritional deficiency responsible for or characteristic of parkinsonism; nor, aside from levodopa, is there any known food or special
nutrient, vitamin, or mineral that has a therapeutic effect. Consequently, there is no dietary treatment. Contrary to what one may
read in magazine articles or popular books on nutrition, there is no
diet or food that is known to have a beneficial effect on the symptoms
of Parkinson's disease or other forms of parkinsonism.

The best dietary advice for patients with parkinsonism is to eat
as normally as possible. The patient should attend to his or her
general health and should eat a well-balanced diet with fruits, veg-
etables, adequate protein, roughage, cereal, etc.

Since a tendency to constipation is common in Parkinson patients,
special attention to roughage and natural laxatives is warranted.
Many patients find it beneficial to eat prunes or figs regularly.
Roughage and "high-fiber" foods are particularly helpful in increasing the bulk of the stool. Patients who tend to have small, hard,
"rock-like" stools should also make an effort to drink more water.
A regimen of four to eight glasses a day to be taken even if one
does not feel thirsty should be followed. Observing these simple,
well-known, effective principles can appreciably reduce the need

for laxatives. Unfortunately, many patients seem to prefer to resort to laxatives than to follow these more natural practices. Thus the best results are found in patients who have a concerned spouse able to encourage, constantly remind, and even scold as needed.

We mentioned earlier that a heavy protein meal such as a hearty steak dinner tends to reduce the absorption of levodopa. If levodopa is taken after such a meal, it is poorly absorbed and the therapeutic effect may be diminished. Some dietitians recommend that patients avoid excessive protein intake and limit themselves to the recommended dietary allowance of 56 grams per day for men or 46 grams for women. This is a very small amount of protein—less than that found in an ordinary one-quarter pound hamburger.

The tendency of protein to interfere with levodopa therapy suggests that low-protein diets might be useful. In fact, such diets have been studied as possible adjuncts to levodopa therapy, and the results are clear: Levodopa is absorbed much better on a low-protein diet— so much so that symptoms of overdosage may occur if the dose is not reduced. A smaller dose yields the same blood level and the same results when the patient is on a low-protein diet as a larger dose when the patient is on a normal diet. Unfortunately, the results are otherwise similar. There seems to be no definite advantage in the low-protein diet. Moreover, since patients find the diet monotonous and tedious, it is not surprising that such diets have been generally abandoned.

The best course is to adjust the dosage to the patient's customary diet, but then the diet should be consistent. Meals should be at regular times. Gastronomic excesses should be avoided.

There is no reason to proscribe the use of alcoholic beverages in normal amounts. Those who are accustomed to having a glass of wine at dinner need not abandon this custom. Patients who enjoy a glass of beer or a cocktail in the evening or at a social occasion need not be deprived of this pleasure. Moderation and common sense are the watchwords here. Excesses should be carefully avoided.

Strangely, alcoholism seems to be very rare among parkinsonian patients. There seems to be something about Parkinson's disease which protects against this all too common scourge. The reason is not known.

In this day of popular dietary foods, "megavitamins," "natural" foods, and health food stores, a few words about these foods in respect to parkinsonism seem in order. Generally, there is no reason the Parkinson patient may not partake of these currently popular dietary fads if he or she so desires. However, there should be no hope that such foods or megavitamins can influence the disease. Some may be "good" in the sense that they are nutritious and thus "good" for anybody, but not specifically for parkinsonians.

Vitamins are substances required by the body in minute or "trace" amounts. Deficiency of the known vitamins can cause serious disturbances. Specific deficiency diseases are known for each vitamin: scurvy results from vitamin C deficiency, beriberi from vitamin B_1 deficiency, rickets from vitamin D deficiency, and so on. If the Parkinson patient has no deficiency and eats a normal diet, taking supplemental vitamins is useless. Contrary to popular belief, vitamins do not supply "pep" or energy or strength. They are taken as a sort of insurance against some possible deficiency due to poor eating habits. It is probably a good idea for older persons generally to take a multiple vitamin tablet daily, especially since the elderly often eat poorly. There is nothing specific about Parkinson patients that makes them susceptible to vitamin deficiencies. However, there is an interesting story about vitamin B_6 (pyridoxine) and parkinsonism which we might do well to review briefly.

THE PYRIDOXINE STORY

Vitamin B_6 was recommended for the treatment of parikinsonism shortly after it was first discovered about 1938. It proved ineffective, and in 1950 the American Medical Association's Council on Pharmacy consulted leading experts on the subject and concluded that pyridoxine had no place in the treatment of parkinsonism. However, pyridoxine is known to be essential for the optimal function of the enzyme that controls the chemical conversion of DOPA to dopamine in the body. For this reason, when the deficiency of brain dopamine in Parkinson's disease was first discovered, there was renewed interest in pyridoxine. It was tried again in the treatment of parkinsonism in large doses: 1,000 milligrams per day or so, approximately 1,000 times more than the daily dose recommended for nutritional purposes. Again, no effect was noted. Nevertheless, the notion that pyridoxine was good for persons with Parkinson's disease persists among some nutritionists, and accordingly they recommend that foods known to be rich in pyridoxine be included in the diet. These include wheat germ, bran, brewer's yeast, tomatoes, liver, and soybeans. Brewer's yeast is very rich in vitamin B_6 and has been recommended for Parkinson patients. These foods are perfectly fine for anyone to eat, and Parkinson patients may certainly eat heartily of them. However, no one has ever presented any evidence that patients eating these foods fare any better than patients who do not. Since pyridoxine, even in doses far larger than the amount available in foods, has been found ineffective in treating parkinsonism, it seems unlikely that foods rich in vitamin B_6 are helpful.

In the early days of levodopa, research physicians added pyridoxine in the expectation that they would thereby enhance its conversion to dopamine. There seemed to be no advantage in doing so. In fact, to everyone's surprise, it proved deleterious. It was found that adding pyridoxine canceled out all the effects of levodopa.

Patients doing well on levodopa who took "therapeutic" vitamins containing large amounts of pyridoxine suffered a gradual recurrence of their Parkinson symptoms within a week or two as if the levodopa were no longer working. When they stopped taking the vitamin pills, the levodopa gradually became effective again.

The reason for this effect of pyridoxine on levodopa treatment is that, in the presence of abnormal amounts of the vitamin, the enzyme which converts levodopa to dopamine does so much faster. It converts it all to dopamine before it can get a chance to reach the brain. Dopamine, alas, cannot enter the brain to reach the dopamine nerve cells of the substantia nigra.

Patients on levodopa treatment should obviously avoid taking pyridoxine or "therapeutic" vitamin tablets containing more than the minimum daily requirement of pyridoxine. The requirement for

vitamin B_6 is not precisely known, but 0.5 to 1 milligram is recommended. This amount does not adversely affect levodopa treatment, but 10, 15, or 20 milligrams per day does. If for some reason
it is advisable for a patient to receive "therapeutic" doses of vitamins,
a special preparation is available under the name Larobec, which
contains all the vitamins in therapeutic doses, *except pyridoxine*. It
was specifically formulated for Parkinson patients on levodopa treatment.

When the pyridoxine reversal of the levodopa effect was first
recognized, some people recommended that patients *avoid* foods
rich in pyridoxine. Diets and lists of foods to be avoided were
prepared and widely distributed. Perhaps there is enough pyridoxine
in concentrated wheat germ to reverse at least partly the benefits of
levodopa treatment. With this exception, however, there is no reason
to avoid foods because of their pyridoxine content. There is not
enough pyridoxine in ordinary diets to affect significantly the metabolism of levodopa. That being the case, there seems no com-
pelling reason to run the uncertain risk of inducing a pyridoxine
deficiency.

The drug carbidopa, which was discussed in Chapter 7, has an
effect opposite to that of pyridoxine: It inhibits the enzyme that
converts levodopa to dopamine. Fortunately, it does not enter the
brain. If it did, it would prevent the formation of dopamine in the
brain and thus prevent the good effects of levodopa treatment. Because of its action, carbidopa should prevent the pyridoxine reversal
of the levodopa effect in parkinsonism—and so it does. Thus patients
on treatment with carbidopa plus levodopa (Sinemet) can eat anything they please and take all the vitamins they wish without risking
"pyridoxine reversal." However, a word of caution is in order. The
protection against pyridoxine reversal may not always be complete.
Thus it would still be wise to avoid "therapeutic" vitamins or "me-
gadoses" of vitamin B_6 unless they are really necessary and prescribed by a physician. Fortunately, there are very few conditions
that require treatment with large doses of vitamin B_6.

VITAMIN C

Ascorbic acid (vitamin C) has enjoyed a popular reputation as a preventative and treatment for the common cold ever since Professor Linus Pauling claimed it was effective in preventing colds. Very large (mega) doses have been used: 0.5- or 1.0-gram tablets one to several times daily. Whether vitamin C is effective in preventing colds need not concern us here. There are, however, theoretical reasons to suspect it might adversely affect levodopa treatment. In practice, only a negligible effect can be discerned, which can be overcome by a slight increase in the dosage of levodopa. There seems to be no reason Parkinson patients may not take vitamin C in any reasonable dose. It might be used, for example, to acidify the urine in cases of bladder infection.

VITAMIN E (ALPHA-TOCOPHEROL)

Vitamin E has been widely promoted as being helpful in an immense variety of conditions. The large number of areas in which it has been claimed to be effective suggests that it is not effective in any. It was reported to relieve painful leg cramps, especially those occurring in sleep (nocturnal cramps). I have given it to a number of Parkinson patients complaining of leg cramps, and I am sorry to say that it did not seem helpful in any. The patients sometimes thought it helped but ceased using it after awhile. Some complained it made them drowsy and tired.

So far as we know vitamin E is relatively harmless, and there seems little reason to object to anyone using it who believes he derives some benefit from it. The recommended dose is one tablet containing 400 international units to be taken at bedtime. Larger doses may interfere with the absorption of vitamin A. Recently, vitamin E deficiency has been found to be the cause of deterioration of peripheral nerves seen in patients with chronic intestinal malabsorption. The symptoms include weakness of the legs, unsteadiness in walking, diminished sensation in the legs, but nothing resembling parkinsonism. In these patients, the blood level of vitamin E is very low.

VITAMIN B$_{12}$

Injections of vitamin B$_{12}$ are sometimes administered by physicians as a sort of "tonic." I have seen patients who claim that it makes them feel stronger. Physicians may give it in the hope of relieving the sense of weakness or fatigue which is so common a complaint in Parkinson patients. However, there is no known reason or clear evidence that vitamin B$_{12}$ injections are indeed helpful in dealing with these symptoms.

Deficiency in vitamin B$_{12}$ results in a particular kind of anemia, termed pernicious anemia. Patients with this disorder have an inability to absorb vitamin B$_{12}$ from the diet. If vitamin B$_{12}$ deficiency is suspected, tests can be done to determine if in fact there is a deficiency. The amount in the blood can be measured. If a deficiency is found, its cause should be determined by appropriate tests, and treatment with vitamin B$_{12}$ instituted. Otherwise, there is no recognized justification for vitamin B$_{12}$ treatment in parkinsonism.

MINERALS

Due to the tendency for bones to lose their calcium content gradually over the years, many physicians and nutritionists recommend supplemental mineral intake for the middle-aged and elderly. There is no evidence that such calcium ingestion really changes the gradual thinning of bones with age. However, within reasonable doses, it does no harm. Similarly, some iron solutions are often recommended, especially to menstruating women, to counter the loss of iron in menstrual blood. Iron deficiency leads to anemia, but in the absence of iron deficiency supplemental iron is useless. Iron deficiency anemia should be treated with large doses of iron, much larger than the amount in the usual vitamin tablet "fortified" with iron. In any event, iron has no therapeutic effect in parkinsonism and does not relieve the sense of fatigue or weakness unless there is indeed an iron deficiency anemia. The physician can easily determine with a blood count if the patient is anemic, and the amount of iron in the body can be determined by sending a tube of blood to the laboratory to measure its iron content. If iron deficiency is present, the doctor can treat it appropriately. If not, there is no need to take iron or iron-fortified vitamins. Iron, incidentally, tends to increase constipation.

Sodium chloride, the mineral sprinkled on food as common "table salt," may be helpful in combating the low blood pressure encountered in some patients on levodopa therapy. The doctor should prescribe the amount. Usually, 1 or 2 grams per day does the trick. This is much more, of course, than can be obtained by salting food heavily. Salt tablets in 0.5- and 1-gram sizes are usually readily available in drug and grocery stores, especially during the summer. There are, however, potential medical complications of excessive salt intake. It may exacerbate high blood pressure, chronic congestive heart failure, and so on. Thus older persons should let their doctor decide if they need to take salt tablets.

AMINO ACID SUPPLEMENTS

The amino acid L-tryptophan has been studied for some years as a treatment for depression. Good evidence has accumulated that in large doses (10 to 15 grams per day) it can indeed relieve the common depression or involutional melancholia of middle age. The dose required is considerably larger than the amount one could get by dietary manipulation. Purified L-tryptophan is now sold in health food stores and is said to be an effective "natural" sedative and tranquilizer.

L-Tryptophan is a naturally occurring amino acid and is a precursor of the chemical messenger serotonin in much the same way that levodopa is the precursor of dopamine. Both dopamine and serotonin are present in the corpus striatum in substantial amounts. The relationships between these two important chemical messengers in the brain is not yet fully understood, but there is some evidence of antagonism. Large doses of L-tryptophan have been reported to exacerbate parkinsonism especially when combined with pyridoxine. L-Tryptophan has also been reported to diminish the severity of chorea, a condition which is in many ways the opposite of parkinsonism. Some clinicians have advocated giving L-tryptophan to patients receiving levodopa to counter the side effects of the latter. I have given L-tryptophan in very large doses to Parkinson patients on levodopa therapy and could find no effect whatever on the parkinsonian state itself or on the side effects of levodopa.

It has been reported in various lay publications that L-tryptophan is beneficial for tremor. Some patients have therefore obtained the amino acid at their local health food store and taken it on their own. It is quite possible the L-tryptophan may be helpful in certain kinds of tremor, such as the severe tremulousness known as action myoclonus, but it is not helpful in parkinsonism.

It is not very clear why one naturally occurring amino acid is regarded as a drug, whereas another, tryptophan, is treated as a harmless dietary supplement that can be bought over the counter. Whatever the logic of this curious situation, I advise Parkinson patients not to use such substances without first consulting their physicians. There are possible problems with dosages, drug interactions, and untoward effects that should be considered.

PHENYLALANINE

Another amino acid some patients obtained in health food stores is the amino acid phenylalanine. They were led to do so by a report in a popular magazine that phenylalanine had been found helpful in treating parkinsonism by a doctor in Buenos Aires. As it happens, I heard the doctor describing his findings at a medical meeting. He had worked with the D-form of phenylalanine. This was very interesting because the late Dr. George Cotzias had found some years ago that giving Parkinson patients L-phenylalanine made them appreciably worse. The doctor in Buenos Aires thought that D-phenylalanine had a different action and was mildly effective in controlling tremor in experimental animals and several patients. He was planning further studies to test its possible value in human patients.

The editors of the magazine that carried the story had not paid attention to which form of phenylalanine had been used. Health food stores do not have D-phenylalanine, only the L-form. The D-form is available only as a chemical reagent at a prohibitively high cost. It does not occur in nature and so must be synthesized. Thus the patients who were experimenting on themselves were using the wrong form of the amino acid! Perhaps that is just as well, because little is yet known of the effects and toxicity of the synthetic D-form of phenylalanine in human subjects whereas the L-form is a normal constituent of the diet. Interestingly, it is converted in the body to tyrosine, an essential amino acid, which was discussed in some detail in Chapter 7.

CHOLINE AND LECITHIN

Dopamine is not the only chemical messenger affected by the ingestion of its precursor. Several years ago Dr. Richard Wurtman and his colleagues at the Massachusetts Institute of Technology showed that the same thing held true for several other chemical messengers. For example, the amount of acetylcholine formed in the brain can be increased by feeding its precursor choline. Practical application of this finding was soon made by various clinical investigators. It was found that supplementing the diet with large amounts of choline chloride, 10 to 15 g daily, could suppress the involuntary movements in certain types of chorea. It was also claimed that choline could at least partially correct impairment of recent memory in some patients afflicted with senile mental deterioration or with Alzheimer's disease.

Many people have been obtaining choline in the form of choline tartrate at health food stores or over the counter at drug stores and chemist's shops in the hope of improving their mental function. Whether it can actually do so in the doses thus used is unclear. None of my patients appear to have enjoyed any benefit. There is a good reason for being cautious about the use of choline in Parkinson patients. In view of the reciprocal seesaw relationship between dopamine and acetylcholine, which we discussed in Chapter

5, one might expect that increasing the formation of acetylcholine in the brain should exacerbate the parkinsonian state. And in fact, it does just that! Therefore, I do not advise my patients to take choline.

One useful source of choline is lecithin. Its full chemical name is phosphatidylcholine. Lecithin is a useful way of administering choline in the treatment of certain types of chorea and especially tardive dyskinesia. It has no place, however, in the treatment of parkinsonism.

CHAPTER 12

Common Sense About Exercise

Physical activity in amounts commensurate with one's ability and strength can make an important contribution to health and well-being. Activity is necessary to maintain the body's musculature. Unused muscles quickly atrophy; similarly, joints need to move through their normal range of motion every day. A joint which is not used soon becomes stiff and eventually suffers a permanent loss of function. The surrounding tissues become firm and fibrotic. The joint can ultimately become frozen in a fixed posture. The patient is then said to have a *contracture* of that joint. Thus constant activity is essential to keep our musculoskeletal system with its muscles, bones, and joints functioning properly. Exercise also improves the heart and the circulation. Increased breathing during physical activity improves aeration of the lungs. The urinary tract, including the kidneys, ureters, and bladder, functions better in the upright position and is thus benefited when the individual rises and moves about. It is a common observation that physically active people have less trouble with constipation than those who lead sedentary lives. Finally, physical activity has a good effect on the mind. It is relaxing, calming, and often provides a welcome change of ideas. A sense of satisfaction and well-being is commonly experienced following exercise.

These obvious truisms merit repetition here because, alas, Parkinson patients tend gradually to withdraw from their usual activities. For various reasons, they seem to do less and less as time goes on and eventually retire to a sedentary existence if a conscious effort is not made to continue normal activities. They seem to suffer an inertia which is probably an expression of the bradykinesia of Parkinson's disease (described in greater detail in Chapter 3). To combat this tendency, it is a good idea to follow a regular routine to assure a reasonable amount of physical activity every day. Whatever the activity, it should be done daily, regularly, and in moderation. Sudden bursts of frenetic activity separated by long periods of indolence are to be deplored. A regular and constant level of activity is best. If this can be done without even thinking about it, if the patient's life style includes a regular and moderate amount of physical activity, that is all to the good. The specific nature of the activity is not important. I am not discussing physical activity as a treatment but as a means of maintaining a degree of physical fitness. No amount of physical activity or specific type of exercise can alter the basic disease process in the nervous system. However, a patient who remains physically fit is better able to cope with the various symptoms of Parkinson's disease as the years go by. It is a matter of common experience that patients who keep physically fit fare better in the long run than patients who do not.

Some patients are fortunate in having an occupation which involves some measure of physical activity. I know a horticulturist who retired at the usual age of 65 years after developing Parkinson's disease. He was able to remain active in his work after retirement working as a consultant and maintaining his own large garden and raising new rhododendron hybrids. The physical activity involved in his work provided him an excellent quality of exercise. This man was also very fortunate in being able to continue after retirement the work he had known and loved most of his life. Some patients have a hobby or avocation which similarly entails some appreciable amount of good physical activity: fishing, hiking, rock collecting, etc. They should by all means continue these activities. How much and how often they can do so is unfortunately often limited by weather, opportunity, and the seasonal nature of some of these activities. One of my patients learned to be an amateur glider pilot shortly before he developed the first symptoms of Parkinson's disease. He was able to continue this hobby for a number of years. Ultimately, he had to give up gliding because of the progression of his disease, but in the meantime he had derived pleasure and satisfaction from it as well as some excellent physical activity. Many patients obtain perfectly good exercise through the pursuit of less dramatic but equally satisfying activities such as tending their gardens, doing light carpentry and masonry, or other yard work around the house.

Obviously, those patients who are able to cultivate an interest in something which keeps both mind and body active are very fortunate. I wish it were possible for more patients to develop such interests. There are so many opportunities for leisure activities today it is a tragedy that more patients seem unable to do so. Unfortunately, most patients have to carry out some program of exercise as a routine chore. It would be much better if it were fun to do, but exercise is sufficiently important that patients should faithfully do some every day as a duty to themselves even if it seems dull. It is a good idea for many patients to have someone else monitor the performance of their daily exercise routine whatever it may be. The patient's wife or husband, relative, or friend should see to it that it is done. The patient may need to be reminded. The monitor should be prepared to urge, coax, or even insist that the exercise be done. Spouses naturally resent the role of drill sergeant, but it is a fact that patients with devoted spouses who see to it that some daily physical activity is done, and done properly, fare much better than those who are allowed to lapse into sedentary and inactive lives, slumped all day before a television set.

Exercise machines, stationary bicycles, rowing machines, and similar devices are very popular, and many patients use them happily and with benefit. However, there is nothing specific about this type of indoor exercise. It is useful when one cannot get more natural exercise. All that is really necessary is to put every muscle and joint through its normal range of motion a few times every day. The exercise need not be intensive or of long duration. It should not be pushed to the point of exhaustion or discomfort.

Walking is an excellent and moderate exercise. The speed, duration, and terrain can be varied to suit the patient's ability and strength. It is not tiring. Indeed, many patients find walking refreshing and relaxing. It is a convenient form of exercise that can be done equally well in the city, suburbs, or country. One can make a point of walking every day in the course of doing certain errands, for example, walking to the corner store to get the newspaper every day. The return walk can be by a circuitous route, perhaps a different one now and then to give some variety. Walking a mile a day is a reasonable and quite common goal. Some patients find this too mild an exercise. Others can walk considerable distances in the pursuit of some hobby. I recall one patient who for many years walked throughout the city of New York to satisfy his interest in historical buildings. Another walked extensively through the fields and woodlands of New Jersey collecting and studying wild flowers. He became something of an expert on the wild flowers of that state. One of my patients is an admitted "physical fitness nut" who jogs every morning. He had been jogging for years before he developed Parkinson's disease, and continued this habit; now, more than 10 years later, he still jogs a mile every morning. This vigorous exercise has no doubt greatly benefited him but I would not routinely recommend jogging to all patients and would not advise it for older patients who are not accustomed to it.

Swimming is also an excellent exercise. Patients who were good swimmers in earlier years may find this a satisfying activity to pursue. Of course, they need regular access to a suitable facility, preferably one available throughout the year. I do not advise a Parkinson patient to undertake to learn swimming for the first time. Also, swimming must be done under adequate supervision. Patients subject to recurrent episodes of bradykinesia may suddenly find themselves in serious trouble in the water should they suddenly freeze and be unable to function. Patients with significant disturbances of equilibrium and walking should avoid water activities. They are likely to have difficulties wading in shallow water and often also have trouble controlling their bodies when swimming in deep water. They may need to be rescued by a lifeguard. It is a cardinal rule of water safety that no one should swim alone. The best of swimmers heed this rule for they realize that they are not immune to having a cramp or some other accident in the water. Certainly Parkinson patients cannot ignore this rule.

Patients who have athletic skills in various sports such as tennis, golf, or squash should continue these activities. Of course they can rarely be done on a daily basis and thus cannot be the only activity used for exercise. However, the pursuit of a learned skill is an excellent way to get healthful exercise. As noted in Chapter 3, learned or acquired skills are apt to be less affected by parkinsonism than automatic instinctive inactivites such as walking. Thus patients who are able to continue a sport of this type requiring considerable motor skill can enjoy a quality of exercise which would otherwise be difficult if not impossible for them to obtain in other activities. If you are already an experienced mountain climber, water skier, acrobat, or what-have-you, by all means continue that activity within reason and safely within your capabilities and the limitations imposed by your parkinsonism.

CALISTHENICS

Some persons have cultivated the habit of doing calisthenic exercises as a daily ritual, usually on arising in the morning or on retiring in the evening. This excellent habit should certainly be continued by those who develop Parkinson's disease. Of course, age and general health are important factors that determine which exercises can be done. Obviously push-ups, skipping rope, or jogging are too strenuous for older persons. Those with a diminished exercise tolerance may do simpler exercises, however, such as bicycling motions with the legs, circling movements with the arms, bending movements, and perhaps even squatting and sitting-up exercises. These various movements may be described as *active range-of-motion* exercises. They assure that every large joint and its related muscles are put through their full range of motion. Repeated 5 to 10 times or more in a systematic way, these exercises can be very helpful in maintaining physical fitness.

I hesitate to recommend any specific set of exercises for so diverse a group of people as the population of Parkinson patients who may come across these pages. However, for the average patient 50 to 70 years of age whose symptoms are reasonably well controlled on proper medical treatment, perhaps the following simple calisthenics may be suggested. Many patients find these too mild and wish to do more. Others may find one or two of these exercises too strenuous or difficult. The patient should consult a physician before embarking on these exercises to be sure there are no medical reasons for not doing them. In any case, these are offered simply to illustrate the type of exercises which many patients find helpful. Usually they are done in the morning on first arising but can of course be done any time. No exercise should be continued which causes pain or discomfort or seems too difficult.

1. While lying flat on your back in bed, slowly lift one leg, knee bent, as high as you can; then straighten the leg until the toes point to the ceiling. Hold this position for 30 to 60 seconds, then slowly lower the leg to the surface of the bed. Repeat 5 to 10 times, first with one leg, then with the other.

2. Lying flat on your back, bend your head slowly to the right to bring the ear close to the shoulder; then slowly bend to the left in the same manner. Repeat 10 times in each direction.

3. Turn over to lie on your abdomen. Place hands behind your back then lift the head, look up to the ceiling and try to lift the chest off the surface of the bed. Now turn your head to the right and to the left, 5 times in each direction.

4. Still lying flat on your back, clasp your hands behind your head and try to sit up. Repeat 5 times. (This may be too difficult for some patients.)

5. Sit up on the side of the bed, feet on the floor, and place hands on hips. Lean forward as far as possible, then lean backward, but do not fall back onto the bed; sit up straight, then lean first to the left, then to the right until the elbows touch the surface of the bed. Repeat 5 to 10 times.

6. Stand up straight with hands on hips, head held high, shoulders

back, and chest thrown forward. March in place 20 steps. Be sure to raise the knees up high and count out loud.

7. Stand erect, raise arms out to side, bringing hands on a level with the shoulders. Then raise arms and bring hands together over your head. Slowly lower arms to the horizontal, pulling the shoulders as far back as possible. Finally, lower arms to the side. Repeat 5 times.

8. Stand erect, then bend forward from the hips in a relaxed manner. Allow the arms to fall downward, your hands hanging limply, fingers pointing to the floor. Do not force yourself to touch your toes with your fingers. This usually happens easily after you have done this exercise a number of times. Stand up straight. Repeat 10 times.

THERAPEUTIC EXERCISES

We have been discussing activities and exercises of a general nature performed with the goal of maintaining physical fitness and which may be useful to anyone, not only patients with Parkinson's disease. There are, however, certain types of exercises that may be done with the aim of helping patients deal with specific Parkinson symptoms, such as stooped posture, the tendency to shuffle on walking, trouble getting up out of deep chairs, or various other difficulties carrying out ordinary tasks of daily life. Ideally, therapeutic exercises should be prescribed by a physiatrist (a physician trained in the medical speciality of physical medicine and rehabilitation) and should be performed by the patient under the supervision of a physical therapy nurse or technician, usually called a physical therapist. Most community hospitals have a department of physical medicine where physical therapy can be obtained on a doctor's referral. For those who are home-bound, periodic visits by a physical therapist to instruct the patient in the exercises can be very helpful. The patient, however, must do the exercises at home alone every day, preferably under the watchful eye of his or her spouse, relative, or friend. Often the patient needs some assistance to perform certain exercises. At the next visit, the therapist can check the progress achieved, see that the patient is still doing the exercises properly, and modify the exercises or suggest new ones as needed. The therapist can reinforce the patient's performance by repeating the instruction and supervising the actual performance of the exercises.

The best exercises are *active* exercises, done by the patient. The role of the therapist visiting the patient at home is mainly to see that the patient knows how to do them and that an appropriate program of activities is being done. If necessary, the therapist can also administer *passive* range-of-motion and stretch exercises which the patient cannot do alone. However, such exercises must be done daily. It is not practicable to have a therapist visit the home daily, so the spouse or someone else must learn to do this type of physical treatment if it is needed. The therapist can teach the technique.

The following exercises are frequently recommended for specific problems. I can only give a few examples here. The therapist can teach additional ones or modify these to meet the special needs and circumstances of each patient. They should be done regularly, every day. They may help only for a short time after each performance, but a cumulative beneficial effect can usually be discerned after weeks of diligently practicing them every day.

Exercises for Stooped Posture

1. Back up against a wall, making sure that heels, shoulders, and the back of the head all touch the wall. Stand in this position for 1 minute, then walk, or better yet, march across the room stepping high and return to the wall. Turn about and back up against the wall again. Note how much you have slumped forward during your march across the room and back. Repeat the entire exercise 5 times in the morning and again 5 times in the evening (Fig. 11).

2. Stand facing the wall, raise your hands as high as possible, and lean forward, placing the palms of your hands on the wall. Slowly push your hands up the wall as far as you can reach, arching your neck and spine backward a little and stretching upward. Repeat 5 times twice a day.

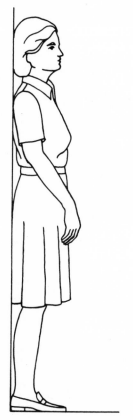

FIG. 11. Exercise for stooped posture.

Exercises for Shuffling and Festination

1. Practice walking or marching with high steps. Count a military type marching cadence and keep time: "hup, two, three, four; left, right, left, right," and so on. Listen to the sounds of your feet striking the floor to get the rhythm.
2. If there is still difficulty raising the feet, place a series of books, magazines, wood sticks, or other objects of similar size in a line across the room about one step apart. Step over these objects in marching across the room (Fig. 12).

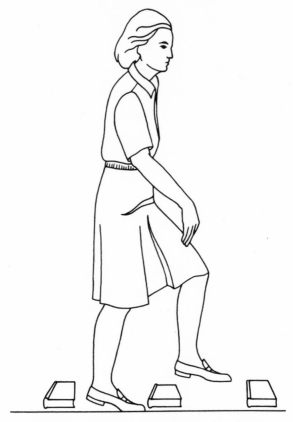

FIG. 12. Exercise for shuffling and festination.

3. When freezing occurs and the feet feel glued to the floor, practice rocking from side to side, swinging the arms and counting a marching cadence out loud. If this fails, stop a moment, think about something else, and then try again. Marching in place for a few steps may also help to break through the "block."

Exercise for Sitting and Rising from Chairs

If you have particular trouble getting up out of chairs, practice sitting down and rising. Use a simple straight-back chair. Study

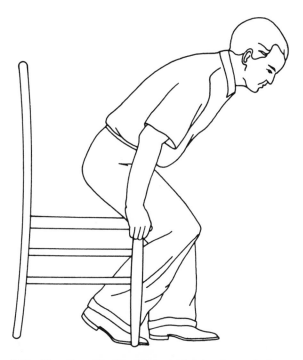

FIG. 13. Exercise for sitting and rising from chairs.

carefully the mechanics of sitting down and getting up out of a chair. To get up, slide forward on the seat, lean forward from the hips so that the trunk is inclined forward approximately 45 degrees, position your feet with one foot under the edge of the seat and the other a half-step forward, and then place your hands on the sides of the seat near the front legs of the chair. Now push and step forward in one continuous smooth motion. If necessary, count to yourself: "one, two, three, GO!" If you fail on the first attempt, rest a moment and try again. Try to get up suddenly before the Parkinson brady-kinesia has a chance to block the movement (see Fig. 13).

To sit down, approach the chair briskly, turn about, then bend the trunk forward 45 degrees and sink down S L O W L Y onto the seat. Be careful to turn a sufficient amount to assure that you end up properly centered on the seat. Try not to fall or slump into the chair. For practice, sit and arise 5 to 10 times. Pay careful attention to each step in the sequence. A common failing is to sit down before turning about fully with the result that the patient sits on one-half of the chair or misses the chair entirely and ends up on the floor. Proper footwork is the key. It helps if one foot is slightly behind the other and directly under the seat.

Speech Exercises

Patients whose speech is difficult for others to understand may benefit from practicing singing and reading aloud. Read the headlines from the daily newspaper, exaggerating the enunciation of each syllable. Sit before a mirror and watch the movements of the lips and tongue while reciting. Go slowly, breathe deeply, and forcefully blow out each syllable separately and loudly to practice projecting the voice. Listen carefully for each consonant and pause between the words. Recite to a measured beat marked by your hand or foot.

Patients are often not fully aware of their speech impairments. There seems to be some defect in their auditory self-monitoring. It may thus help to practice speaking into a tape recorder. Listen as you play back the phrase or newspaper headline you have just recited. Do it again, trying to correct the deficiencies you heard. By repeating this several times at one sitting you will find that it is possible to improve speech function to a considerable degree.

If speech impairment is a major problem, ask your doctor to refer you to a qualified speech therapist.

Miscellaneous

Making faces before a mirror helps to maintain the mobility of the facial muscles. Grin, frown, smile, snarl, pout, whistle, and puff out the cheeks.

If chewing and swallowing food is a problem, make an effort to chew first on one side, then on the other. Note the sound of the teeth while chewing; maintain the rhythm. Swallow small, well-chewed morsels only. Avoid the common habit of quickly swallowing half-chewed food.

SENSORY REINFORCEMENT

You may have noticed that in these various exercises I stressed the importance of sensory stimuli. Counting out loud a marching cadence, using visual cues to guide the feet, and rocking from side to side to provoke stepping are all means of enhancing the sensory stimuli with which we normally although unconsciously monitor motor performance in complex activities. Consciously adding strong stimuli addressed to sight, hearing, and the sense of the body's position in space serves to reinforce the normal physiological mechanisms underlying the performance of complex motor acts such as walking, talking, getting up out of a chair, and so on. This sensory reinforcement is a useful principle in physical therapy, especially in the therapy of Parkinson patients. Patients can learn to make effective use of it in many circumstances, each in his own individual manner. Many of my patients have discovered this principle by themselves. One patient controlled his drooling tendency by constantly keeping a piece of raw carrot in his mouth. Its mere presence served to stimulate an increased frequency of swallowing and thus prevented the excessive accumulation of saliva in the mouth which might then overflow as drooling. Another patient had nails placed in the heels of her shoes. She listened to the resulting "click clack" as she walked. She found that it made her conscious of the rhythm of her walking and prevented episodes of festination which had been troubling her gait. Many patients have discovered other similar tricks that have helped them function better.

The principle of sensory reinforcement is employed in the formal physical therapy of Parkinson patients with good effect. Walking exercises, for example, are done in a group session with a number of patients to the beat of a drum. Calisthenics are similarly done in a group to the accompaniment of music with a strong rhythmic beat.

TIPS FOR PROBLEM SITUATIONS

Patients having particular trouble with their equilibrium on walking should have more formal gait training exercises under the supervision of a physical therapist, preferably in a properly equipped physical medicine facility. Several suggestions have often proved helpful. First, consider shoes. If the patient suffles he or she will probably do better in shoes with leather or hard-composition soles. Shoes with rubber soles, especially crepe rubber, may be more comfortable to wear but cannot easily slide on most surfaces. Consequently when you shuffle with a soft rubber sole, your foot is likely to stick to one spot and cause you to lose your balance and fall.

Patients who tend to step backward a few steps involuntarily (retropulsion), and are thus subject to falling backward, may benefit from wearing shoes with heels. A heel lift inside the shoe may also help. Slippers with flat heels or no heels tend to increase the tendency to retropulsion. On the other hand, patients who have more difficulty with propulsion (that is, falling forward) may do better on low or flat heels. Scatter rugs and mats are an additional hazard for patients who shuffle. It may be a wise precaution to remove them from the home. Door sills may also be a problem, since freezing and festination indoors occur particularly at doorways. If necessary, door sills can easily be removed by a carpenter.

Patients who have trouble getting out of chairs should learn to avoid deep, upholstered chairs, especially those with low seats and soft cushions. Try to choose instead straight-back wood chairs, preferably with arm rests, such as the traditional "captain's chair." Remember the exercise described above for getting out of chairs. Be sure to move forward to the edge of the seat, position the feet for proper leverage, and push up with both hands, leaning forward as you get up. If the patient needs help getting up from a chair, merely holding his or her hand and providing slight support may suffice. The mere contact of the hand seems to provide a necessary reference point. The sensation seems more important that the actual force or support provided. If that does not do the trick, the patient's companion may then place one hand on the patient's head and push forward gently but firmly. As the patient then tries again to get up, he may exert considerable back pressure against the companion's hand; however, the patient nearly always can rise briskly. Very little pressure is usually required. I usually can help even patients who have great difficulty getting up with the pressure of one finger. It is much easier to help the patient in this way than to stand in front and pull him up and forward by the hands. The latter procedure may sometimes be needed, but one must be careful; the patient can be pulled up to standing only to fall on top of his helper, with both patient and companion ending up on the floor.

Reclining chairs can be obtained with a spring-loaded lever-actuated seat which pushes the patient up and forward on arising. Some patients find these chairs very helpful, but those with poor equilibrium may have difficulty. As they are pushed up and forward, they must be able to step forward. Patients who have difficulty standing and stepping forward may instead fall forward. I strongly advise a patient contemplating the purchase of such a chair to try it out first and be sure that it is actually helpful.

A simpler trick is to have the rear legs of the patient's favorite chair raised 5 or 6 centimeters (approximately 2 inches) with blocks or a crossbeam. This gives the seat a slight forward tilt which makes it easier for the patient to get up and yet does not make the chair less comfortable.

A cane provides less support to the Parkinson patient with a walking problem than might be expected. Even walkers are often disappointing. The patient with poor balance and subject to episodes of retropulsion simply falls backward—cane, walker, and all. Canes can be helpful to the patient with propulsion, and many patients do learn to use them effectively. Four-legged canes are helpful to patients with poor equilibrium. There are many varieties of canes and walking aids, and the patient should be trained in their proper use by a physical therapist. The therapist can also ascertain what type of device will be most helpful.

The patient with severely impaired walking and poor equilibrium, and who is subject to frequent falls, may nevertheless have very good stepping movements and be able to walk well providing he is accompanied by someone who can catch him in time to prevent a fall. Such a patient should have a brief daily walk with someone in attendance as a form of exercise.

Attention to the disposition of furniture around the house helps prevent injuries in case of falls. There should be an adequate rail on stairways. Hand bars on the wall near the bathtub and toilet should be installed. The toilet seat can be raised an inch or two with blocks. A chair can be placed in the shower stall or in the bathtub to render bathing easier and safer. Rubber bath mats should help reduce the chance of falls in the bathroom.

Those patients who have difficulty dressing, buttoning clothes, tying shoes, etc. due to lack of fine control of finger movements may benefit from several modifications of their clothing. Where possible, zippers or patches of adhesive cloth can be used instead of buttons. Polo shirts or T-shirts may be used in place of front-buttoned shirts. Shoelaces may be replaced by elastic laces that do not need to be tied or untied. "Loafers" or similar "slip-on" shoes without laces may be even more comfortable.

REHABILITATION SERVICES

Most patients need only practice a simple regimen of exercises on their own or with the help of their families to maintain a normal amount of physical activity. Some patients may, in addition, benefit from the occasional assistance of a physiatrist and a program of physical therapy with exercises along the lines of those just discussed. A small number of more severely affected patients who have problems carrying out the ordinary activities of daily life may need more intensive physical therapy in order to prevent invalidism. If the symptoms of Parkinson's disease become so severe, despite good medical treatment, that the patient can no longer manage to live independently at home, whether alone or with his or her family, then perhaps admission to hospital or to a special rehabilitation unit for a thorough evaluation and a more intensive course of physical therapy may be indicated.

A patient who has deteriorated more rapidly than expected deserves a complete medical evaluation to make sure that some other disease process is not complicating the scene. The first indication that something else is going on—an ulcer, a kidney infection, a cancer, or some other serious illness—may be an unexpectedly rapid decline over a period of months in a patient who was formerly doing quite well in controlling the symptoms of Parkinson's disease. If something is found, it may be possible to correct it and restore the patient to his or her former health. Perhaps nothing serious will be found, but revision of treatment in a hospital setting may prove beneficial. Intensive physical therapy while in the hospital is usually an important part of such treatment.

In hospital, physical therapy can be given daily for several hours at a time. Every aspect of the patient's performance of daily living activities can be reviewed. Special training can then be given to teach the patient ways of overcoming the disabilities imposed by parkinsonism, and to eat, dress, bathe, comb, brush, and do the numerous ordinary tasks of daily life. In addition, intensive physical therapy can improve the patient's gait, posture, equilibrium, and performance of various motor acts.

When the patient returns home, every effort should be made to continue some physical therapy at home to maintain the benefits gained in the hospital for as long as possible. The program of exercises must be carried out daily. A visit every week or two to the physical medicine department at the hospital serves to check progress and review the home exercise program. If necessary, arrangements can often be made to have a physical therapist visit the patient at home. The therapist may be able to make useful recommendations regarding the patient's life at home, the installation of hand rails and grab bars, and the use of various self-help devices. It may also be advisable to obtain some help at home. A part-time attendant or "home health aide" may be necessary to help the patient and family cope with the invalidism of advanced Parkinson's disease. The goal is to try to keep the patient at home and as independent as possible for as long a time as possible. The periodic visits of the visiting nurse service, if there is one in the area, may be very helpful. The visiting nurse can give valuable advice, help make arrangements for physical therapy, transportation to the doctor's office or clinic, and provide home health aides and other medical social services.

Unfortunately, it is often difficult to convince the "third party" organizations such as the medicare carriers, medicaid, and other health insurers to pay for physical therapy and other services at home for patients with chronic diseases. They do not seem to mind paying for such care to a patient recovering from a fracture or a stroke who needs therapy for only a limited time, but they are very reluctant to commit their funds and personnel to a course of therapy which may need to be continued indefinitely. They do not seem to understand that providing limited services at home such as a weekly visit of a physical therapist and a visiting nurse is in the long run a great deal better for the patient and a lot less expensive than the alternative of chronic care in a nursing home.

CHRONIC CARE FACILITIES

Ultimately the patient with far-advanced Parkinson's disease may become too great a burden for the family, and at that point placement in a nursing home or chronic care hospital must be considered. Each case, of course, is different and must be evaluated on its individual merits. Some families are able to set up what is in effect a nursing home at home with hospital equipment, private nurses and attendants, and so on. Most families, however, lack the resources—personal, emotional, and economic—to pursue such a demanding course. Moreover, it is not necessarily the best course for the patient. It is rarely possible to reproduce all the services and quality of care at home that is provided by the better nursing homes. For many patients rendered invalid by severe parkinsonism, a nursing home is preferable. Before making the final decision to seek nursing home placement, the patient and family will probably meet with a medical social worker.

Usually contact with a medical social worker is first made in hospital at the request of the patient's doctor. The social worker here provides an essential service. The worker can review with the patient, the spouse, or other relative assuming responsibility for the patient's needs the doctor's recommendations and the prognosis. Applications to suitable homes can then be initiated. The spouse or other responsible person should, if possible, visit the various facilities being considered. In most areas there is a substantial waiting period for admission to a chronic care facility. It may be 2 to 3 months or more before a vacancy is likely to open up in a desirable home. Thus the patient may have to go home for a time to await admission to the nursing home of his or her choice.

Among the things to consider in choosing a nursing home is the availability of good physical therapy. Is there a suitably equipped physical therapy facility? Are full-time physical therapists employed? Can bedside therapy be given if needed? In even the patient with the most far-advanced case of Parkinson's disease who is confined to bed and chair, physical therapy can offer much relief of discomfort and help with specific troublesome symptoms. Active and passive movement of the limbs, training in the fine art of using a wheelchair to full advantage, and ambulating with support if necessary can all make significant contributions to the patient's comfort and general well-being at this stage of the disease.

In summary, exercise has a definite place in the management of Parkinson's disease at every stage in its evolution. The choice of type of activity is a highly individual matter to be decided in consultation with the treating physician. In earlier stages of the disease informal exercise and physical activity intended to maintain physical fitness are important. The problems which arise with more severe disease can be mitigated by specific exercises. Later, more intensive physical therapy may be required. Finally, even in the most advanced stages of the disease, great benefit is provided by physical therapy. Indeed, it is in the later and more severe stages of the disease that physical therapy can make its greatest contribution. If I may be permitted one final word of advice to Parkinson patients on this general subject, it is this: Never give up any activity, never give up an inch of your independence until you absolutely must, for it is much more difficult to regain a lost activity than to hold onto it a little longer with the aid of some judicious exercise or physical therapy.

CHAPTER 13

A Historical Perspective

Our present understanding of parkinsonism did not spring into being overnight but grew gradually over a long period of time, very slowly at first and then more and more rapidly. Most of our knowledge was gained during the last 15 years. It has grown and changed appreciably even during the last few years. Doubtless it is changing even as I write this passage and will surely continue to change during the years ahead. It is not possible to give a final version of the truth about parkinsonism. It is not even possible to give the illusion that we can do so at this time, in the last quarter of the 20th century, because our knowledge and our concepts of the brain are evolving very rapidly. For this reason alone it is helpful to review briefly the history of our knowledge of parkinsonism so as to place present concepts in some perspective.

The modern history of parkinsonism may be said to have begun in 1817 when James Parkinson published a small monograph entitled *An Essay on the Shaking Palsy*. In its pages we find the first clear description of the condition we now call Parkinson's disease. The description is admittedly incomplete. Parkinson, a physician and surgeon practicing in London, had seen six cases over a period of some time. He was able to examine only one. It must be remembered here that the physical examination carried out by the modern medical practitioner had not yet been developed. None of the clinical techniques needed for evaluating the nervous system were then known. Neither the stethoscope nor the reflex hammer were yet in use.

Moreover, the modern reader finds Parkinson's literary style quaint and archaic. Nevertheless, his account is remarkable for its accuracy and clarity of expression. In a few words, he cut right to the heart of the matter. His opening chapter begins with the following terse yet comprehensive definition.

"Shaking Palsy (Paralysis Agitans): Involuntary tremulous motion, with lessened muscular power, in parts not in action and even when supported; with a propensity to bend the trunk forwards, and to pass from a walking to a running pace; the senses and intellect being uninjured."

Some of the symptoms mentioned in this definition had been described long before. Indeed, the ancient Greek-Roman physician Galen wrote of tremor of the hand at rest and distinguished it from a tremor occurring during movement. That is, Galen made a distinction between a resting tremor and an action tremor. It is thus tempting to believe that Galen knew of Parkinson's disease but we cannot be certain because he does not associate the tremor with the other symptoms. Similarly, the "tendency to pass from a walking to a running pace" had also been described long before Parkinson's time. Indeed Parkinson himself referred to a description rendered by the 18th century French physician Sauvages, who had termed the abnormal gait *sclerotyrbe festinans*. On reading Sauvages' account, one feels that he had very probably seen cases of Parkinson's disease. Yet, since he did not mention any other symptom, we cannot be certain.

Goethe, the great German poet, had some medical training. He noted that the innkeeper in Rembrandt's sketch of "the Good Samaritan" stands in a stooped posture holding his hands before him with the thumbs opposing the fingers as if counting coins—or as patients with Parkinson's disease often do (Fig. 14). Goethe commented that the artist had been so skillful that the innkeeper's hands actually appear to tremble. One wonders if Rembrandt had intended to represent a case of Parkinson's disease, by whatever name (if any) it was known in his time. It is tempting to believe that so acute an observer as the great artist undoubtedly must have seen cases we would now call Parkinson's disease; but again, we cannot be certain.

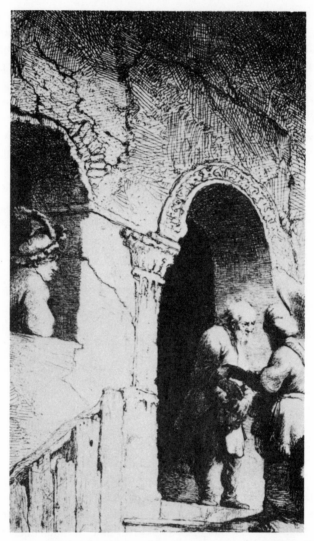

FIG. 14. The Good Samaritan in Rembrandt's famous etching. The poet Goethe thought the innkeeper seemed to have tremor of the hands. The man's appearance is suggestive of Parkinson's disease.

There are other hints that Parkinson's disease has been with us a very long time. However, the possibility that James Parkinson was describing a truly new disease cannot be dismissed. A major problem is that the art of medicine was not sufficiently advanced prior to James Parkinson's time to provide much light on the subject. Very few diseases were known in their entirety. Every symptom was described as an independent entity unto itself. Medical writing was replete with descriptions of symptoms but not of entire patients. It was only toward the end of the 18th century that combinations of symptoms came to be recognized as expressions of specific diseases that had a beginning, a particular pattern of evolution, and a termination, and hopefully could be explained by, or at least correlated with, anatomical changes to be found on postmortem examination. The early 19th century was a time when many of the diseases known today were first described and a beginning was made at correlating the symptoms present in life with changes found on postmortem study. Many of these diseases bear the names of the early medical writer who first described them. Thus we have from the early 19th century not only Parkinson's disease but also Bright's disease, Hodgkin's disease, Bell's Palsy and so on. In many cases the names of the early describers have been dropped and more descriptive names have been used. In a few cases, however, no satisfactory term has been found, and so the eponym (the name of the physician who first wrote about the disease) remains in common use. Thus it is with Parkinson's disease. No satisfactory descriptive term has been found. The original term "shaking palsy" seems too vague. Its Latin translation "paralysis agitans" is no better, although it may sound more "scientific" merely because it is Latin. Diseases that were first identified from postmortem studies are often designated by terms describing the essential pathological findings. Thus we have among nervous system disorders such entities as spinocerebellar degeneration, striatonigral degeneration, and olivo-pontocerebellar atrophy. Conceivably we might describe Parkinson's disease as substantia nigra atrophy, but that is only one of the anatomical changes found in the brain and fails to convey a picture of the complex pattern of symptoms that is yet rather characteristic. More-over, Parkinson's disease was fully recognized by its signs and symptoms long before its pathology was identified, so that the name Parkinson's disease has been established by a long and continuous usage. There seems to be no good reason to change the name at the present time. It seems appropriate to commemorate the history of our knowledge of the disorder in its name.

Parkinson deserves recognition for having "connected" the several symptoms he noted and for having recognized that patients at "different stages of its progress" were victims of the same disorder. This was an important contribution and a considerable accomplishment in his time. We must grant Parkinson full credit for having been the first to recognize the shaking palsy as a specific morbid entity in its own right.

Many other physicians contributed to our knowledge of Parkinson's disease. One especially deserving mention was Jean Marie Charcot, a great medical teacher of the mid-19th century and one of the founders of modern neurology. Charcot studied patients with the shaking palsy and considerably enlarged Parkinson's description. He added the muscular rigidity and many other manifestations. In 1867 he introduced treatment with the alkaloid drug hyoscine derived from the plant *Datura stramonium*. Drugs of this type remained the mainstay of treatment until the advent of levodopa a full century later. A scholarly man with a keen interest in history, Charcot insisted that the shaking palsy should be named Parkinson's disease because Parkinson had been the first to describe it and because the term shaking palsy seemed inappropriate. There was, he argued, no true paralysis or palsy as in the case of stroke, for example, and some patients had no tremor.

One of Charcot's students, Paul Richer, was also an artist. He is best remembered today for a textbook on human anatomy he wrote for artists (which has recently been translated into English by Robert Hale). His sketches of Charcot's patients at the Sâlpétrière hospital in Paris are classics of medical illustration and were widely reproduced in medical textbooks of the latter 19th century. One of his sketches is shown in Fig. 15.

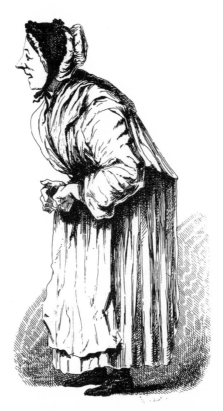

FIG. 15. Sketch of patient Anne Marie Gavr.... at the Sâlpétrière hospital in Paris drawn by Paul Richer in 1874.

As a result of the work of Charcot and other medical teachers, during the latter 19th century Parkinson's disease became a well-recognized disorder. It seems fair to say that physicians of the 1890s were as familiar with it as physicians are today.

Parkinson had been able only to speculate on the cause of the disease and on the location of the disturbance in the nervous system. He expressed the hope that "those who humanely employ post-mortem anatomical examination in detecting the causes and nature of diseases" would be able to ascertain its "real nature" so that "appropriate modes of relief, or even of cure" might be found.

Many physicians engaged in studying the pathology of nervous system disorders sought to find the nature of the disease as Parkinson had hoped. Their labors, however, were for a long time unproductive, and there was much speculation regarding the site of the trouble in the brain. Some thought the problem was in the spinal cord, and others thought it was in the muscles; but mostly no consistent abnormality could be found. Parkinson's disease was thus classified for a time as a "neurosis," meaning thereby that there was no known structural change in the brain to explain the symptoms. In short, there was an obvious disturbance of function without an apparent material cause. One can readily see on reading discussions of the disease written during the 1890s that this was a perplexing and frustrating state of affairs.

One of Charcot's students, Professor Brissaud, suggested that the place to look for the material basis of Parkinson's disease might be in a certain small nucleus or nerve center in the brainstem, the substantia nigra. Studies of this area of the brain were later made postmortem. There was great difficulty distinguishing changes that might be due to aging, arteriosclerosis, or the disease itself. Finally, a student named Tretiakoff working on his doctoral thesis in Paris described a number of changes in the nerve cells of the substantia nigra which are now recognized as typical of Parkinson's disease. His thesis was published in 1915, nearly a century after Parkinson's *Essay on the Shaking Palsy*. These findings were not readily accepted by the medical scientists of that time. Many neurologists were skeptical that injury to so small a group of obscure nerve cells could give rise to all the varied symptoms of parkinsonism. Others thought that loss of nerve cells in other areas, especially in the corpus striatum, was a more likely cause of the symptoms. Controversy continued on this subject for many years.

The recurrent epidemic of sleeping sickness, or encephalitis lethargica, which struck during the years 1916–1926, brought great confusion to the whole subject. Rather suddenly neurologists were confronted with large numbers of relatively young patients having symptoms bearing some resemblance to those of Parkinson's disease. There were also some striking differences. The victims of this new disease were relatively young, mostly between the ages of 15 and 30, whereas previously parkinsonism under age 40 had been extremely rare. Suddenly the young parkinsonian patient had become commonplace in the neurological clinics and wards of big city hospitals. These young patients had many bizarre symptoms that had never before been associated with parkinsonism. There was no question that parkinsonism following encephalitis lethargica was a new and different disease.

The recognition that there could be two kinds of parkinsonism soon led to the labeling of other conditions that bore some resemblance, however remote, to Parkinson's disease as types of parkinsonism. Thus there came about the notion of arteriosclerotic parkinsonism and parkinsonism due to carbon monoxide or other chemical intoxications. The various entities became confused—so much so that during the 1930s some physicians began to suspect that all parkinsonism was due to encephalitis! A more popular view was that there was no such thing as Parkinson's disease, but that "parkinsonism" was simply a fortuitous grouping of symptoms reflecting many different diseases. With the concept of parkinsonism in such a confused state, it is not surprising that pathologists had difficulty confirming Tretiakoff's findings. Moreover, progress was hampered by a lack of knowledge about the substantia nigra and the corpus striatum.

The structural changes in the brain in cases of encephalitis lethargica were studied and defined. Here too the substantia nigra was consistently found to be affected, and it was thought that perhaps this change was related to the Parkinson symptoms. Then a German pathologist, Dr. R. Hassler, studied in exhaustive detail the substantia nigra in Parkinson's disease and confirmed the earlier findings of Tretiakoff. His work was published in 1939, but because of the disruption of World War II it received little attention for some years. After the war the noted brain pathologist Dr. J. G. Greenfield studied the brains of parkinsonian patients at London's famous National Hospital for Nervous Diseases, and further confirmed the constant involvement of the substantia nigra in Parkinson's disease. Gradually, more and more brain pathologists came to agree that here was the major site of anatomical derangement in Parkinson's disease.

The significance of the changes observed in the substantia nigra remained obscure for a long time. No one knew what the substantia nigra did or how extensive its connections were with other brain regions. Research anatomists tried to injure the substantia nigra in animals but were unable consistently to produce manifestations similar to those of human parkinsonism. There were considerable technical difficulties, and no one was quite sure how a parkinsonian cat or dog or monkey should look.

A major step forward came with the demonstration, using a new microscopic technique developed in Sweden, that the nerve cells of the substantia nigra contained the chemical substance dopamine. The new technique depended on a chemical reaction which changes dopamine into a substance that shines brightly green when placed under ultraviolet light. A brilliant group of young Swedish researchers including Drs. Urban Ungerstedt, Anita Dahlström, Kjell Fuxe, and Nils-Erik Andèn applied this technique to the rat brain and demonstrated whole systems of nerve cell pathways that had previously been unknown. Among these was an important system of fibers that arose from the nerve cells of the substantia nigra and went to all areas of the corpus striatum. This new discovery in the field of brain anatomy was given additional meaning by new discoveries in other areas. Biological chemists found that dopamine was present almost exclusively in these two regions of the brain. One researcher, Oleh Hornykiewicz, working in the Medical School of the University of Vienna, measured this substance in the brains of patients who had died with various diseases and found that dopamine was strikingly deficient in those who had parkinsonism but not in those with any other disorder. On further work he found that the dopamine deficiency was greatest in those cases in which the pathologists found the most severe changes in the substantia nigra.

Related research in animals showed that when the substantia nigra was injured dopamine disappeared from the corpus striatum on the same side. This indicated that there must be a connection between the substantia nigra and the corpus striatum, and provided further evidence of the existence of the pathways the Swedish scientists were finding in the rat with their new technique. This was important because these fibers could not be demonstrated by the classic methods of brain anatomy. Brain anatomists were skeptical at first; but as this sort of evidence gradually accumulated and was confirmed by other workers in research laboratories in other countries, the existence of the dopamine nerve cell system gained acceptance.

In the meantime a third key observation had been made by Professor Arvid Carlsson at the University of Göteborg in Sweden. In 1957 he carried out a simple experiment that clarified the way in which reserpine produced its tranquilizing effect. As indicated in Chapter 1, reserpine is a major tranquilizer that can produce in man a condition closely resembling Parkinson's disease. Chemical measurements had shown that reserpine caused depletion of various substances in the brain, including noradrenaline, dopamine, and serotonin. Some thought that the tranquilizing effect was due to the depletion of serotonin. Professor Carlsson found that an injection of levodopa immediately reversed the tranquil state that had been produced in the animals by reserpine, whereas the precursor of serotonin did not. He also measured the amount of dopamine in the brains of the animals and found that the levodopa had restored the dopamine levels to normal.

These various discoveries achieved independently in separate scientific fields were certainly interesting and important in themselves. In combination, however, they gave a new meaning to the changes in the substantia nigra first found in Parkinson patients by Tretiakoff a half-century earlier and explained the production of parkinsonism by the tranquilizing drugs. Parkinsonism could now be defined as a state of brain dopamine insufficiency. Professors Carlsson and Hornykiewicz both suggested that levodopa might be tried as a treatment for parkinsonism.

Thus James Parkinson's hope that postmortem anatomical examination might reveal the "real nature" of the "shaking palsy" has been at least partially fulfilled. The location of the dysfunction in the nervous system responsible for the major symptoms is now known. We also have a general idea of the type of disease process involved, although the exact cause remains unknown. Most important, an "appropriate mode of relief" based on this knowledge is now available.

These discoveries, which so greatly clarified the nature of parkinsonism, came chiefly during the decade 1957–1967. However, they represented the culmination of many decades of scientific research and thought. They could not have been achieved, say, during the 1930s or 1940s because the basic knowledge of brain chemistry was lacking. Indeed, even the fundamental techniques—such as the use of radioisotopes and the analytical techniques in organic chemistry which made the measurement of dopamine and related substances in the brain possible—were unknown prior to 1950. Thus it is that practical advances in medical care depend on the state of science as a whole, and that so-called "pure" research in basic science having no obvious connection to practical problems leads eventually to profound new understanding of human disease and entirely new forms of treatment.

Initially levodopa was given in small doses by injection into a vein or in small doses by mouth. The first physicians to try levodopa were Dr. Walter Birkmayer of Vienna and Dr. Andre Barbeau of Montreal, Canada. Many others soon attempted the same approach. There was marked disagreement among various investigators regarding the results. Some reported dramatic improvement even in severely affected patients. Others found no effect at all, and still others noted some minimal improvements but thought they might be due to psychological factors, such as the enthusiasm of the investigators rather than to the levodopa effect. There were a number of investigators who thought there were definite effects but concluded that the results were too limited to be of practical value for the treatment of Parkinson patients.

Then Dr. George Cotzias, a medical scientist working at the Brookhaven National Laboratories in Upton, New York, found that much larger doses by mouth yielded better results. He found that if he continued to administer DOPA (at first he worked with a 50–50 mixture of D-DOPA and L-DOPA or DL-DOPA) every day for weeks and months, the patients gradually became tolerant of the side effects. Nausea and vomiting gradually diminished and disappeared, so that progressively larger doses could be given. By persisting patiently, raising the dose every few days as his patients slowly developed a tolerance for DOPA, Dr. Cotzias was able eventually to give doses 20 to 30 times larger than the initial dose. With very large doses (as high as 12 to 18 grams of DL-DOPA per day), he obtained striking improvements in patients with typical and quite severe parkinsonism. The effects of DOPA were clearly much greater than those attainable with the conventional anti-Parkinson drugs previously available.

Dr. Cotzias first reported his results with DL-DOPA in 1967. Within a year they were confirmed at several other research centers. A large, carefully controlled study conducted by Doctors Melvin Yahr, Margaret Hoehn, Robert Barrett, Myrna Schear, and myself at the Columbia-Presbyterian Medical Center in New York helped gain acceptance of levodopa administration as a normal treatment for Parkinson's disease. Large-scale clinical trials of levodopa were then undertaken under the sponsorship of two pharmaceutical firms (Hoffmann-LaRoche and Eaton Laboratories) to evaluate the safety and efficacy of levodopa under the conditions of ordinary medical practice.

Several thousand patients were treated under research protocols at major teaching hospitals and medical research centers throughout the United States and in many other countries. Levodopa was consistently found to be more effective in the treatment of parkinsonism than any other treatment then known. It was so effective in comparison to the drugs previously in use that the stereotactic surgical procedures widely used at that time for parkinsonism were largely abandoned almost overnight. The generic name levodopa was chosen for the medical preparation of L-DOPA as a drug. It was formally approved by the Food and Drug Administration (FDA) for use in treating parkinsonism in 1970.

L-DOPA was a major advance in the medical treatment of diseases of the nervous system. The principle it represents—administering the metabolic precursor of a chemical messenger substance deficient in the brain in a certain disease—has since been extended to other disorders with some success. Probably the major importance of levodopa was that its very success stimulated great interest among neuroscientists in the study of Parkinson's and related diseases, and opened up new and promising directions for future research that may lead to still more effective treatment.

Looking back over this brief historical perspective, one can see that our present understanding of parkinsonism has grown steadily from a small, inconspicuous beginning more than a century and a half ago. We can also see how this growth was a part, a small part to be sure, of the extraordinary growth—one might perhaps better say "explosion"—in our knowledge of the structure and function of the nervous system and its dissolution in disease that has taken place over the past century. The growth is continuing at an accelerating pace, so we may expect that our understanding of parkinsonism and the underlying brain dysfunction will continue to grow at a rapid pace during the years ahead.

CHAPTER 14

Future Prospects

The future holds real promise of a better life for patients with Parkinson's disease and their families. How soon and to what extent this promise will be realized depends primarily on the successes achieved during the years ahead in fundamental research in the nervous system. This field of research is alive today and rapidly advancing. Never before have so many talented investigators devoted so great an effort to studying the development, structure, and function of the brain. Many anticipate that major advances will be made during the next 5 to 10 years. Recently Dr. Donald Tower, director of the National Institute for Neurological Diseases, Stroke, and Communicative Disorders, predicted that the next 10 years will be "the decade of neuroscience." The result will be greater understanding of many currently obscure neurological disorders including Parkinson's disease. In fact, patients with Parkinson's disease seem especially likely to benefit, for their disease is a major focus of current research.

The success of levodopa therapy has greatly stimulated interest among scientists in areas of biological science relevant to parkinsonism. Much effort is now devoted to exploring the normal structure and function of those areas of the brain particularly affected. The metabolism of levodopa and the chemistry of the dopamine nerve cell is the subject of many studies. Research is under way into the growth and development of the substantia nigra and the corpus striatum, as well as into their decay during senescence.

Postmortem studies of the brains of persons who have had various types of parkinsonism are providing new insights and changing our concepts of the nature of Parkinson's disease. Such studies paved the way to the use of levodopa as a treatment and may be expected to contribute to the development of new therapeutic approaches once again in the future. Studies in animal models of parkinsonism are providing a better understanding of the mechanisms of action of the treatments currently used and offer strong promise of improving them. They may also tell us something about the kinds of change that occur in the brain when the substantia nigra deteriorates, and how we may help the brain compensate for the loss of the dopamine nerve cells. Animal studies currently in progress should lead to a better understanding of the nerve cell systems specifically affected and of their special susceptibility to various metabolic poisons which may normally be formed in the body.

We may be reasonably confident that these lines of scientific attack will lead to still better treatments for Parkinson's disease and related disorders. We also hope that they will uncover clues to the ultimate cause of Parkinson's disease and thus to a truly curative treatment. One must be realistic, however, and recognize that there is no immediate prospect of finding the cause this year or next. Nor can we even anticipate from which area of research the critical clues may come. It is possible, of course, that someone may inadvertently stumble on the answer next month; indeed many if not most major advances in science have come from unexpected or accidental discoveries. This is called serendipity. However, we cannot plan for or count on a serendipitous discovery. We can only hope that the more good people we have working on a problem, the more likely such a discovery may be. Moreover, we must hope that the critical clues will be recognized when they are observed.

Pending a serendipitous "breakthrough," we must patiently pursue the path of increasing our fundamental knowledge of the nervous system. We need to know much more than we do now before we can reasonably expect to find the cause and cure of disorders such as Parkinson's disease. It is not merely a matter of spending a sufficient amount of money and effort. The necessary fundamental knowledge simply does not yet exist.

A wealthy man afflicted with Parkinson's disease once asked me to mount a "crash program" of medical research to find a cure for the disease quickly. He hoped we could emulate in medical research something like the spectacular success of the Apollo Space Program. The situation we face, however, is quite different from that which confronted the scientists of the space program. The necessary fundamental knowledge in physics, astronomy, and engineering was already available. All that was required was to apply the theoretical knowledge at hand. An enormous amount of money, talent, and effort was able within a few years to place men on the moon. The neuroscientist of today is concerned with gaining that essential body of theoretical knowledge. It may well be achieved during the decade ahead providing fundamental research receives the financial, moral, and administrative support it needs.

Medical research today is dependent chiefly on the financial support of the federal government administered by the National Institutes of Health in the form of research grants, contracts, and fellowships. Grants on a much smaller scale are also provided by some pharmaceutical firms, but these are usually given to help defray the costs of running clinical drug trials. An additional but limited source of funds to support research is provided by private philanthropic gifts and small grants from private foundations. Notable among these are the Parkinson's Disease Foundation of New York, the United Parkinson Foundation in Chicago, The National Parkinson Foundation in Miami, The Parkinson Foundation of Canada in Toronto, and The American Parkinson Disease Association in New York. Small regional societies formed by patients and their families have been primarily engaged in providing aid, advice, and various services to patients. The private foundations do not have anything like the resources of the National Institutes of Health, but they can provide necessary help in critical areas and influence national research policy. They also provide patients an opportunity to express their own views and needs, and to participate in the battle against parkinsonism.

In addition to the fundamental research we have been discussing, there are many active programs of research proceeding at a more practical level into means of improving present methods of treatment and to developing new treatments. New drugs offering promise of better control of symptoms are continuously being tested in clinical drug trials, and others are in earlier stages of development. Let us temper enthusiasm with a word of caution. As the levodopa story so well illustrates, it takes a long time for a new treatment to develop from an idea in the laboratory to a drug doctors can prescribe for their patients.

New drugs usually derive from research in a pharmacology laboratory in a medical school, a university medical research center, the research department of a pharmaceutical firm, or other comparable facilities. If a substance shows promise in an animal model of parkinsonism, it is then considered for trial in human subjects. Before it can be given to humans, permission must be obtained in the United States from the Food and Drug Administration (FDA). (In other countries, permission is sought from similar governmental regulatory agencies.) The sponsor of the proposed new drug, usually a pharmaceutical firm, must provide evidence of safety. Studies must be carried out in animals to assess possible toxicity. Initially, the FDA grants a permit for limited evaluation of the effect of one or two doses in normal volunteers. Data are thus gathered on the doses required and tolerated, the nature of the side effects, and the metabolism of the drug. On completion of those studies, the sponsor may then apply for permission to carry out a trial in patients with the disease or symptom for which it is hoped the drug may be useful. Usually the sponsor is restricted to a small number of patients and a short period of drug administration. For example, the FDA may grant permission to treat 20 patients for 2 to 4 weeks only. The approved protocol requires a battery of laboratory tests to detect any possible toxic effects on the liver, kidneys, heart, and other organs. A common requirement is a weekly blood count and routine urinalysis, blood chemistries before and after the trial, electrocardiograms, and repeated examination of the subjects. In many instances the patient must be admitted to hospital or to a special research unit for the duration of the trial. Usually several such trials are conducted at various facilities by different teams of investigators.

If the new drug passes these preliminary clinical studies satisfactorily and still shows promise, the sponsor may then ask for permission to carry out further trials on a larger scale to test the new drug under conditions similar to those prevailing in ordinary medical practice. A number of physicians expert in the condition for which the drug is a proposed treatment are then invited to try the new drug in some of their patients. Again, a protocol specifying the laboratory tests and outlining the methods of drug administration to be used must be strictly followed. The protocol approved by the FDA defines criteria for establishing the diagnosis and selecting patients for the trials. Patients who have other serious illnesses are usually not accepted for an experimental drug trial because if they suddenly became ill it would be difficult to know whether they were suffering from a side effect of the new drug or an exacerbation of their illness. Patients accepted for an experimental drug trial must also be able to communicate their subjective experiences accurately. Patients with mental illness or serious neuroses obviously make poor subjects. Also, it is usual to select a group of patients with different symptoms in order to test the drug's efficacy fairly against each symptom and in different clinical situations.

The clinical investigators who carry out drug trials are usually faculty members of medical schools or staff members of university hospitals or clinics who have accepted a responsibility for teaching and research in clinical medicine. Drug trials are rarely conducted in community hospitals or private doctors' offices. Each investigator must file a biographical sketch with the FDA and must be specifically approved by the FDA for each trial. He must maintain clinical records of each patient on the trial and a strict account of the drug received and dispensed. Every tablet or capsule must be accounted for. Periodic reports must be filed with the sponsor. Any adverse reactions must be immediately reported on special forms provided for the purpose by the FDA. FDA inspectors make periodic audits of these records.

A properly conducted clinical trial may last several years. Individual investigators may be allowed to subject 40 to 50 patients or more to the new treatment. If the new drug is effective and appears promising, investigators often come under pressure from anxious patients and their families who have read or heard news accounts of the new drug.

Reports of clinical experiments with new drugs are presented each year by physicians engaged in such work at various scientific meetings. Often reporters for newspapers, trade publications, or wire services hear such a presentation and report it on the radio or in a newspaper or magazine. Usually the more favorable and enthusiastic reports are selected by the news media, whereas more critical or sober assessments presented by other investigators at the same meeting are ignored. The result can be misleading, such as the uncritical news account shown in Fig. 16.

I was a participant at the scientific meeting in question and can vouch that the researchers said nothing of the kind. Unfortunately, many patients read a similar item in their local newspaper, or their friends or relatives sent them a clipping. Many weeks later the same account appeared again, in various weekly and monthly periodicals, notably magazines sold at food stores, and in trade publications.

Parkinson's Disease Cure Believed Near

By R. MICHAEL PATTERSON
LUBBOCK, Tex.
Researchers studying Parkinson's disease believe they are close to finding a cure for the chemical normally found in the brain.

"I feel we are on the threshold of an important step and so patients should know that the search is continuing to

FIG. 16. Newspaper account of a scientific report.

This sort of thing goes on all the time. I have seen clippings of similar newspaper accounts printed 30 to 40 years ago! Almost every week a patient brings me a news account of this type hoping that it might contain some truth. Sometimes the patient laughs, for he or she has already been taking the drug for many months and can readily see the discrepancy between reality and the enthusiastic news report. Often, unfortunately, patients are disappointed to learn that the new "miracle" drug is not available or is still an experimental drug that can be given only under research conditions. Many patients, I am sorry to say, are too eager to volunteer to take an experimental drug despite the fact that its potential dangers are yet unknown and that it has many side effects.

The uncritical accounts of a new treatment appearing in the news media cause much mischief. They raise false hopes and spread confusion among patients and their families. These reports must be read critically and skeptically. Patients and their families should by all means ask their doctors about such items. Often the doctor may not know of the research in question, but he may be able to find out about it and describe it to the patient at the next visit. I would also advise patients to call or write to the newspapers or magazines and ask for more details. Perhaps some feedback from the people affected may cause the news media to behave more responsibly in reporting such news.

Unfortunately, the practicing doctor may not read about a new drug in his professional journals until many months after the patients have read about it in their newspapers. The reason is that reporters attending a scientific meeting file their reports the same day, but the investigator presenting a report before his colleagues at that meeting may not submit it to a publisher for another month or two, and the professional journal involved may not be able to publish it for another 6 to 8 months.

The cost of developing new drugs for treating parkinsonism is very great and beyond the means of most medical research centers. Only large pharmaceutical manufacturers are normally equipped to carry out the kind of chemical and biological studies required by the FDA and to prepare chemical agents that can meet governmental purity standards. The costs of carrying out the necessary clinical trials are considerable, and these are usually supported by financial grants from the sponsoring firm, from the National Institutes of Health, or sometimes by private foundations or wealthy patrons. Since most drugs which reach the stage of large-scale clinical trials ultimately fail to make the grade either because of insufficient efficacy or unexpected toxicity, the economics of new drug development are risky and forbidding. It is not surprising that few pharmaceutical firms are willing to venture into the field of parkinsonism.

Despite these obstacles, several new drugs are currently under clinical investigation and a number are in still earlier stages of study. It is very difficult to predict the future, and I do not claim to have a crystal ball, but it may be of some interest to briefly review these drugs and the implications of some current research.

DOPAMINE RECEPTOR AGONISTS

The recent discovery that there are at least two types of dopamine receptors has obvious implications for the search for more effective treatments. The two receptors have been labeled the D-1 and the D-2 receptors, respectively. They are distinguished by differences in chemical properties. They are distributed differently throughout the nervous system. For example, the dopamine receptors in the pituitary gland are of the D-2 type. The corpus striatum contains both D-1 and D-2 receptors. It is not clear yet whether these appear on different nerve cells in the striatum, but there is some evidence that they serve different functions.

One may well ask which receptor is important for the relief of parkinsonism or whether perhaps both are important but relate to different symptoms. These and many other questions await further study. It is already possible, however, to use in animal models, drugs that are selective for one or the other type of dopamine receptor. These new drugs do not yet have names but are identified only by code numbers. For example, there is SKF 39387, which is a highly selective D-1 agonist. Experiments in animal models of parkinsonism carried out by Dr. Gershanik and Dr. Heikkila at Rutgers Medical School have shown that a selective D-1 agonist produces somewhat different effects from those produced by a selective D-2 agonist and that using both together results in a better effect than either alone. A curious aspect of the D-2 agonists is that they do not reverse the Parkinson-like state produced in animals by reserpine. Neither will the D-1 agonist. But both used together yield an excellent reversal. There is also some suggestion that certain side effects may relate mainly to activation of the D-2 receptor. Selective D-1 agonists have not yet been tested in human patients. Hopefully they will be tested soon.

Where current research on dopamine receptors and their agonists will lead us is difficult to predict, but it seems clear that we are likely to see a continuing stream of new, more selective, and more potent agonist drugs in the years ahead. It also seems reasonable to expect that some of them will be more effective than those presently available for clinical use.

DIHYDROXYPHENYL SERINE

It is now clear that norepinephrine as well as dopamine is deficient in the Parkinson brain. However, we do not know what symptoms, if any, result from this deficiency. One symptom might be the tendency of Parkinson patients to have low blood pressures. Perhaps it might relate to changes in sleep patterns. It has also been suggested that norepinephrine may play a role in the control of walking. Thus, some means of replenishing norepinephrine stores may be useful. Treatment with levodopa may at least partially restore brain norepinephrine stores.

Recently, Professor Narabayashi of Tokyo, has reported that small doses of a synthetic amino acid, dihydroxyphenyl serine (DOPS), has beneficial effects on the gait disturbance in certain patients. DOPS is converted directly to norepinephrine, bypassing dopamine. Thus DOPS is a more effective way of replenishing brain norepinephrine stores. Further work with DOPS is awaited with great interest.

DEPRENIL

A drug that inhibits the enzyme monoamine oxidase only in the brain and does not act in the heart or on the adrenal gland has been tried in the treatment of parkinsonism, especially in Europe. Since its action is restricted to the brain, it should enhance the desired effects of levodopa without carrying the risk of provoking hypertension and abnormal heart rates. This drug, deprenil, was initially used in combination with levodopa by Dr. Walter Birkmayer in Vienna, Austria. Other investigators soon confirmed Dr. Birkmayer's reports of a gratifying enhancement of the beneficial effects of levodopa. However, other investigators have not agreed that it is useful. Dr. Donald Calne and his associates at the National Institutes of Health in Bethesda, Maryland, carried out a careful study of deprenil and did not find it more effective than a matching placebo tablet. My own experience with deprenil led to the conclusion that adding deprenil to an existing levodopa regimen is essentially the same as increasing the daily dosage of levodopa by about 20%. Although the theoretical considerations underlying the use of this new drug are attractive, the actual benefits obtained with it in practice seem to be limited.

BRAIN TRANSPLANTS

One of the most fascinating possible approaches to parkinsonism now under study is based on research presently underway in several centers on the transplantation of dopamine-forming nerve cells into the brain. It has been found possible to transplant nerve cells forming dopamine, epinephrine, and norepinephrine from one animal to another, or from an animal's own adrenal gland to its brain. Moreover, such transplanted cells are capable of producing lasting functional effects, such as, at least partially correcting experimentally-induced parkinsonism. The transplanted nerve tissue is placed in one of the ventricles of the brain adjacent to the corpus striatum or injected directly into the corpus striatum. It is theoretically possible to do the same to human Parkinson patients. Indeed, researchers at the

the same to human Parkinson patients. Indeed, researchers at the famed Karolinska Institute in Stockholm, Sweden have already done two transplant procedures in human patients. No formal report of their observations has yet appeared, and so one cannot evaluate the benefits in these patients. It will certainly take some time and more patients before even tentative conclusions can be drawn.

A number of fundamental problems in the underlying cell biology need to be resolved to place the technique of transplantation on a firm basis. It is still not clear what kind of cells would be best, precisely where to put them, whether at one site or many sites, and what volume of tissue to transplant. One might ask whether too much tissue could be transplanted? The simplest procedure would be simply to remove a wedge of tissue from one of the patient's own adrenal glands and place it within one of the ventricles of the brain against the side of the corpus striatum. A small piece of the adrenal medulla, the portion of the gland containing epinephrine, would be used. The medulla contains specialized nerve cells which form dopamine, epinephrine, and norepinephrine as noted on page 83. Transplanted to the brain, these cells appear to form a sort of biological reservoir storing and releasing dopamine, epinephrine, and norepinephrine, which then diffuses into the adjacent corpus striatum. Clearly, this does not restore things to normal, but it could represent a significant improvement for the patient. Which patients would be helped by such a procedure remains to be determined.

In the experimental work that has been done so far, chiefly in rats, it has been found that the adrenal cells, which normally do not have processes, now develop such processes once transplanted into the brain. These processes grow into the corpus striatum for a short distance from the transplant and resemble normal nerve cell processes. It is not known whether human adrenal medulla cells would be able to do the same thing. If they did, there might be some prospect of developing something like normal connections with the nerve cells of the corpus striatum. It has not yet been established, even in the rat, whether these transplanted nerve cells do make connections.

Much more research needs to be done. Yet, although it seems like science fiction, the transplantation of nerve cells into the brain is technically feasible and offers great promise for the treatment of many disorders, including Parkinson's disease. I should not be surprised to see such transplantation surgery being done more frequently in Parkinson patients a decade hence.

CONTINUOUS INFUSIONS OF LEVODOPA

Several groups of investigators have shown that constant infusion of levodopa into a vein can smooth out the fluctuations in patients with a severe degree of the "on-off" effect. At least it seems to do so for 1 day. Some investigators have found that dyskinesias develop on the 2nd day. Thus, it appears possible that some form of "levodopa pump," similar to the insulin pump, which has been used in managing brittle diabetics, may have a place in treating parkinsonism. Many technical problems need to be worked out before such an approach may become practical. Levodopa could not be used because it is so insoluble in water and very acid, but some compound, which could release levodopa, might work, or some other drug might serve the purpose. The technology is available, however, and one can expect continuing efforts to develop drugs and pumps for sustained infusion treatment.

APPENDIX 1

Drug Finder

The most commonly prescribed anti-Parkinson drugs are listed in Tables 1 and 2 (pp. 182–183) with a brief description of dosages and formulations. In addition, see the drawings of the different tablets and capsules marketed in the United States and their identifying marks and numbers (pp. 184–185). I have not shown the generic equivalents, but usually these are produced in plain white tablets or capsules. The same drugs may be produced in different shapes and colors in different countries, often under different names. If there is any doubt about the identity of a forgotten bottle of pills, discard it or consult a pharmacist before using the drug.

Most tablets and capsules have distinctive markings, coloring, and code numbers to facilitate identification. The letters and numbers are often very small, and a magnifying glass may be needed to read them. The manufacturers impress or print an identifying trademark on their products. Lederle Laboratories, for example, has an L in script on the front of each tablet. Tablets are usually scored on the reverse side so that they can easily be broken in half for smaller doses. The 2-mg Cogentin tablet is double-scored and thus can be broken into 0.5-mg fragments.

TABLE 1. *Commonly prescribed anti-Parkinson drugs*

Brand (trade) name	Generic name	Formulations
Anticholinergics		
Artane	Trihexyphenidyl	2 and 5 mg white tablets and 5 mg long-acting capsules
Tremin	Trihexyphenidyl	2 mg white tablet
Kemadrin	Procyclidine	2 and 5 mg white tablets
Pagitane	Cycrimine	1.25 mg orange and 2.5 mg brown sugar-coated capsules
Akineton	Biperiden	2 mg white tablet
Cogentin	Benztropine	0.5 and 2 mg round white tablets and 1 mg long elliptical white tablets
Symmetrel	Amantadine	100 mg bright red capsule
Parsidol	Ethopropazine	10 and 50 mg white tablets
Antihistamines		
Benadryl	Diphenhydramine	25 and 50 mg pink and white capsules
Disipal	Orphenadrine hydrochloride	50 mg round light green tablet
Dopamine receptor agonists		
Parlodel	Bromocriptine	2.5 mg tablets and 5 mg capsules, caramel and white

TABLE 2. *Levodopa preparations*

Larodopa	Pink tablets*
	0.1 gram (elliptical, scored)
	0.25 gram (round)
	0.5 gram (oblong, scored)
	Capsules
	0.1 gram (pink and scarlet)
	0.25 gram (pink and beige)
	0.5 gram (pink)
Dopar	Capsules only
	100 mg (small, opaque green)
	250 mg (medium size, opaque green and white)
	500 mg (large, opaque green)

Levodopa-decarboxylase inhibitor combinations

Sinemet (carbidopa/levodopa)	Elliptical tablets
	10/100 mg (dark dapple blue)
	25/250 mg (light dapple blue)
	25/100 mg (yellow)
Madopar (bensarizide/levodopa)	Capsules
	25/100 mg (pink and blue)
	50/200 mg (caramel and blue)

*Note: 0.1 gram = 100 mg; 0.25 gram = 250 mg; and 0.5 gram = 500 mg.

ANTICHOLINERGICS

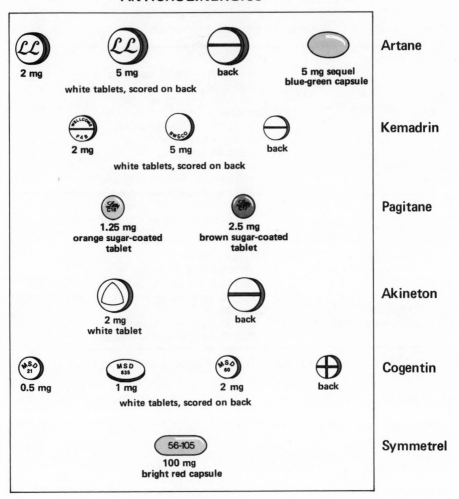

Artane

2 mg 5 mg back 5 mg sequel
blue-green capsule

white tablets, scored on back

Kemadrin

2 mg 5 mg back

white tablets, scored on back

Pagitane

1.25 mg
orange sugar-coated
tablet

2.5 mg
brown sugar-coated
tablet

Akineton

2 mg
white tablet

back

Cogentin

0.5 mg 1 mg 2 mg back

white tablets, scored on back

Symmetrel

56-105
100 mg
bright red capsule

ANTIHISTAMINES

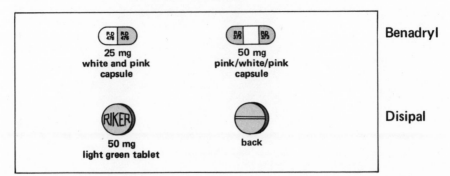

Benadryl

25 mg
white and pink
capsule

50 mg
pink/white/pink
capsule

Disipal

50 mg
light green tablet

back

ANTIHISTAMINES (contd.)

2.5mg tablet

5 mg white and caramel capsule

Parlodel (bromocriptine)

LEVODOPA PREPARATIONS

0.1 gram pink

0.25 gram pink

ROCHE label on back

0.5 gram pink

Larodopa tablets

0.1 gram pink and scarlet

0.25 gram pink and beige

0.5 gram pink

Larodopa capsules

100 mg opaque green capsule

250 mg opaque green and white capsule

500 mg opaque green capsule

Dopar

LEVODOPA-DECARBOXYLASE INHIBITOR COMBINATIONS

10/100 mg dark dapple blue

25/250 mg light dapple blue

scored on back

25/100 mg yellow

Sinemet (carbidopa/levodopa) tablets

25/100 mg pink and blue

50/200 mg caramel and blue

Madopar (bensarizide/levodopa) capsules

APPENDIX 2

Organizations Concerned with Parkinson's Disease

NATIONAL INSTITUTES OF HEALTH

Much of the credit for the great advances achieved in Parkinson's disease in the 1960s and 1970s must be given to the National Institute of Neurological and Communicative Disorders and Stroke (NINCDS) in Bethesda, Maryland. NINCDS is one of the National Institutes of Health, the major United States government agency engaged in medical research, and a part of the Department of Health and Human Services. For many years the NINCDS has maintained a large-scale program of research grants to universities and research laboratories throughout the country, in addition to having an active program of research at the Clinical Center in Bethesda. The Clinical Center is a large medical research facility operated by the US Public Health Service. A small number of patients who live in the Washington, D.C. area are accepted there for experimental drug trials upon referral by their private physicians.

An informational pamphlet on Parkinson's disease may be obtained by writing the Superintendent of Documents, US Government Printing Office, Washington, D.C. 20402. Currently this is DHHS Publication No. (NIH) 80–1616 entitled *Parkinson's Disease*. The cost is $2.25, including shipping.

The NINCDS also makes available an annual summary of research in parkinsonism, prepared each January. A copy may be obtained from the NINCDS, Building 31, Room 8A-06, National Institutes of Health, Bethesda, Maryland 20014.

Many lay voluntary agencies have been active for some years in providing information to patients and their families, educating the public, and supporting medical research. In the United States, there are no less than five major organizations operating at a national level, plus 50 or more local and regional groups. Voluntary agencies have also developed in Canada, Japan, the United Kingdom, Italy, Germany, South Africa, and in other countries. Many of these organizations sent representatives to the International Congress of Neurological Sciences held in Kyoto, Japan, October 1981, to form an International Federation of Parkinson Societies. I do not have the space here to list all these organizations, but will list the five major agencies now active in the United States and Canada.

The American Parkinson Disease Association, Inc.
116 John Street
New York, New York 10034

The Parkinson's Disease Foundation
William Black Medical Research Building
640 West 168th Street
New York, New York 10032

National Parkinson Foundation, Inc.
1501 Ninth Avenue NW
Miami, Florida 33136

United Parkinson Foundation
220 South State Street
Chicago, Illinois 60604

The Parkinson Foundation of Canada
Suite 232 ManuLife Centre
55 Bloor Street West
Toronto, Ontario, Canada M4W 1A6

The *American Parkinson Disease Association*, founded during the early 1960s has for a number of years provided patient advisory services in the New York area and funds to support research projects aimed at improving the treatment of parkinsonism. Most of the financial support was given to the New York Hospital-Cornell University Medical Center in New York City. The medical director, Dr. Fletcher McDowell is a well-known authority on chronic neurologic diseases. He helped develop levodopa therapy. Recently the Association embarked on a national program supporting clinic and information centers scattered throughout the United States. It also issues a quarterly newsletter to bring patients news of recent advances in treatment. Patients may obtain excellent and well-illustrated booklets from the Association, including one describing a program of exercises to be done at home and another outlining various aids and adaptive equipment for home use and a manual for patients. The Association awards small "seed money" grants to help young investigators interested in working in Parkinson's disease research in a number of centers throughout the country. It has also awarded substantial fellowships, the George Cotzias fellowships, to support promising young scientists for 1 to 3 years.

The *Parkinson's Disease Foundation* was established in 1957 by William Black for the purpose of supporting scientific research into the cause of Parkinson's disease with the hope of eventually finding a cure or a means of prevention. The Foundation has supported major international symposia on parkinsonism. It awards research grants and fellowships to promising scientists in the United States and Canada, and supports a program of summer fellowships for medical and other graduate students interested in biological problems relevant to Parkinson's disease. The Foundation also supports a "brain bank" at the College of Physicians and Surgeons of Columbia University in New York. The "bank" consists of specimens of brains removed from Parkinson patients postmortem and a registry of patients who have contributed their remains for research. This is an exceedingly valuable research resource, and patients who desire to bequeath their brains for such research should write to the Foundation about the necessary procedures.

The *National Parkinson Foundation* was established in 1957 by the late S. Jay Levey in Miami, Florida. It has devoted its energies primarily to maintaining and operating an outpatient treatment facility in Miami. It has enjoyed the support of Bob Hope and other show business people. Diagnosis, treatment, physical therapy, and rehabilitation services are provided at this facility to ambulatory Parkinson patients. The "National" Foundation does not currently maintain a residential facility or provide inpatient services. Nevertheless, patients often travel to Miami to receive treatment at its facility for periods of several weeks or more. Recently an affiliation was arranged with the University of Miami School of Medicine. The Foundation has also provided research grants to investigators and has sponsored several international symposia on the treatment of Parkinson's disease. Useful informational pamphlets on the disease may be obtained by writing directly to the Foundation.

The *United Parkinson Foundation* was founded in Chicago in 1963 by Edgar N. Greenebaum, Jr., primarily to provide patients and their families with the knowledge needed to understand Parkinson's disease. Through its regular newsletters, exercise booklets, and other literature, recent developments in research are reported, clarifying reports of new therapies and their efficacy. Beginning with a series of symposia in Chicago, the Foundation has sponsored semi-annual patient-education meetings throughout the country. The speakers are usually drawn from the organization's highly qualified Medical Advisory Board. The executive director of the United Parkinson Foundation, Judy Rosner, regularly attends both national and international neurological meetings, and may be found at the United Parkinson Foundation booth each year at the annual meetings of the American Academy of Neurology. She maintains a high visibility for Parkinson's disease among the community of neurologists and neuroscientists, with the goal of stimulating interest and concern among young scientists. The Foundation is funded by contributions from the general public, with nearly three-quarters of its income now being used to support research grants to established scientists whose primary interest is Parkinson's disease. Fellowship grants have also been made available to promising students working under the direction of specialists in basal ganglia research. Questions and requests for literature may be sent to the Foundation's office in

Chicago. Patients and their families may write to obtain a personal response to specific problems and for referrals to competent clinical neurologists throughout the North American continent. Through its affiliation with the Parkinson's Disease Research Center at Rush-Presbyterian-St. Luke's Medical Center in Chicago, patients wishing to donate brain tissue for research studies may be assisted in the correct procedures by the Foundation's staff.

The Parkinson Foundation of Canada was founded in the 1960s to provide service to patients and raise funds to support research. In 1979 it established a Parkinson Professorship at the Playfair Neurosciences Unit of the University of Toronto at the Toronto Western Hospital. In July 1982, the foundation made 11 grants totaling $200,000 to scientists throughout Canada. A network of local chapters and self-help groups has been developed, which provides therapy, educational meetings, and discussion sessions to help patients and their families cope with the disease. Educational materials including books, tapes, and informational pamphlets are made available to members and the public. The foundation also publishes a regular bulletin.

LOCAL PATIENT ASSOCIATIONS

Many local groups, societies, and associations have been formed by patients and their families with the view of exchanging ideas and sharing advice on means of coping with practical problems. These self-help or support groups have sprung up in recent years in every major city and many smaller cities and towns throughout the United States. Examples include the Dallas Area Parkinson Society, The Parkinson Society of Greater Washington (PSGW) in Washington, D.C., The Parkinson Association of the Rockies in Denver, Colorado, and the numerous Parkinson Education Programs. The PSGW hosted a national convention of Parkinson support groups in August 1981 at Camp Maria, Maryland. Over 50 local support groups were represented. There were also representatives of similar groups from Canada, Mexico, and other countries; some from as far away as Japan and New Zealand. From this meeting there emerged a national organization, The Parkinson Support Groups of America, based in the offices of the PSGW. The Parkinson's Educational Program has also become a national organization with local PEP groups in many cities.

Many of the support groups and local associations publish newsletters for their members, hold regular meetings, provide exercise sessions, and other activities. They provide valuable assistance to patients and their families. Some groups have also raised funds to support the research programs on parkinsonism at various medical schools. They thus provide their members an opportunity to participate directly in the conquest of Parkinson's disease.

Glossary

Adrenaline (also known as **epinephrine**): The hormone of the adrenal gland. It is secreted into the circulation in moments of crisis and stimulates the heart to beat faster and work harder, increases the flow of blood to the muscles, causes an increased alertness of mind, and produces other changes to prepare the body to meet an emergency.

Angina pectoris: A characteristic pain in the chest felt as a squeezing or pressing behind the breastbone. It arises in the heart muscle usually during some activity and subsides with rest. It is a symptom of coronary arteriosclerosis or arteriosclerotic heart disease. The pain occurs when the heart muscle, as a result of impaired blood flow in the coronary arteries, fails to receive sufficient oxygen to carry on the work it is called on to do. Pains in muscles of the shoulder and chest are sometimes confused with angina pectoris.

Acetylcholine: The chemical messenger released by the cholinergic nerves, such as the vagus nerve.

Anticholinergic: Adjective applied to drugs opposing the action of acetylcholine.

Antihistamine: Term applied to drugs opposing the actions of histamine and commonly used to treat allergic disorders such as hay fever and bronchial asthma.

Alpha-tocopherol: Chemical name for vitamin E.

Athetosis: Involuntary movements, which are similar to but slower than chorea; they are usually writhing movements of the hands or feet.

Bradykinesia: Word meaning slowness of movement (derived from the Greek *brady*, meaning slow, and *kinesia*, meaning movement; a cardinal sign of Parkinson's disease.

Benign essential tremor: A condition characterized by tremor of the hands, head, voice, and sometimes other parts of the body which often runs in families. It is sometimes called *familial tremor*, and in the elderly *senile tremor*. It is sometimes mistaken for Parkinson's disease although there is no rigidity or bradykinesia.

Choline: A naturally occurring substance which is a precursor of acetylcholine.

Corpus striatum: Anatomical term meaning, literally, "the striate body" designating a large mass of gray matter deep in each cerebral hemisphere. Its internal structure and function are not yet well understood, but it is believed essentially to modulate or regulate motor and sensory activities of the brain.

Chorea: Diagnostic term derived from the Greek *choriea*, meaning dance. It is applied to a nervous affection marked by excessive motor activity ranging in severity from restlessness, fidgetiness, and twitching to flinging movements, sudden jerks, and spasms; it is sometimes associated with mental agitation. It is popularly known as St. Vitus' dance.

Dopa: Chemical short or "nick" name for dihydroxyphenylalanine, an amino acid occurring in animals and plants. It exists in two forms, the L- and the D-forms. Only the L-form occurs in nature.

Dopamine: Substance derived from DOPA in certain nerve cells. Dopamine functions in the nervous system as a chemical messenger transmitting impulses from one nerve cell to the next. It is deficient in Parkinson's disease.

DOPA decarboxylase: Enzyme found in the nervous system and blood vessels. It controls the metabolic conversion of DOPA to dopamine.

Decarboxylase inhibitor: A drug which inhibits or prevents the action of the enzyme DOPA decarboxylase and thus hinders the conversion of DOPA to dopamine.

Dyskinesia: A general term meaning an abnormal involuntary movement.

Dystonia: A type of involuntary movement, which is slow, twisting, and associated from forceful muscle contractions or spasms.
The painful end-of-dose foot cramp is a common example.

Encephalitis: Inflammation of the brain (from Greek *encephalon*,
meaning brain, and the suffix *itis*, meaning inflammation, as in
tonsillitis, appendicitis, etc.) usually caused by a virus infection.

Encephalitis lethargica: A specific kind of encephalitis which occurred in scattered epidemics throughout the world during the
period 1916 to 1926; it usually caused somnolence, double vision,
trouble swallowing, and drooling in the acute phase, and a special
type of parkinsonism in its chronic phase. The disorder was also
called *von Economo's encephalitis* and *epidemic encephalitis*.

Festination: Walking in rapid, short, shuffling steps (from Latin
festinare, to hasten).

Glaucoma: Disorder of the eye characterized by a sustained increase of pressure within the eyeball which can injure the optic
nerve and cause impaired vision.

Lateropulsion: An involuntary stepping or staggering to one side;
it occurs as a symptom of inflammation of the inner ear and also
of Parkinson's disease.

Lecithin: A naturally occurring substance containing phosphatidylcholine. It may be taken by mouth for the purpose of providing
choline to the nervous system to increase the synthesis of the
chemical messenger acetylcholine.

Levodopa: The international generic name for the medicinal formulation of L-DOPA (L being short for *laevo*, Latin prefix meaning left). The full chemical name is L-3,4-dihydroxyphenylalanine.

Livido reticularis: A purplish or bluish mottling of the skin seen
usually around the knee and sometimes on the forearm in patients
under treatment with the drug amantadine.

Micrographia: The small handwriting characteristic of many Parkinson patients.

Oculogyria: Spasm of eye muscles causing eyes to look upward involuntarily (rarely downward). It has a sudden onset and may last for minutes to hours; it is a characteristic symptom of post-encephalitic parkinsonism following encephalitis lethargica and sometimes occurs as a reaction to certain tranquilizing drugs, but it is never seen in Parkinson's disease.

On-off effect: Descriptive term used to refer to sudden changes in the clinical state of Parkinson patients on levodopa therapy.

Parkinson's disease: That form of parkinsonism originally described by James Parkinson: a chronic, slowly progressive disease of the nervous system characterized clinically by the combination of tremor, rigidity, bradykinesia, and stooped posture, and pathologically by loss of the pigmented nerve cells of the substantia nigra.

Parkinsonism: A clinical state characterized by tremor, rigidity, bradykinesia, stooped posture, and shuffling gait. The more common causes of parkinsonism are Parkinson's disease and a reversible syndrome induced by major tranquilizing drugs.

Paralysis agitans: The Latin form of the older, popular term "shaking palsy," which was used to designate Parkinson's disease in James Parkinson's time. It is currently the official diagnostic term for Parkinson's disease of the World Health Organization's International Statistical Classification of Diseases.

Phenothiazines: A class of drugs extensively employed in medical practice for various purposes. One group includes anti-histaminic agents (e.g., Phenergan) and anti-Parkinson drugs (e.g., ethopropazine), and another larger group comprises the major tranquilizers (e.g., chlorpromazine), which can induce a Parkinson-like state.

Paradoxical kinesia: Sudden, usually brief episodes of marked remission of symptoms of parkinsonism which may last minutes, sometimes hours, and rarely several days.

Paresthesia (plural: paresthesias): Sensations, usually unpleasant, arising spontaneously in a limb or other part of the body, variously experienced as "pins and needles" or a feeling of warmth or coldness (thermal paresthesias).

Palilalia: A symptom of parkinsonism, especially the postencephalitic form, in which a word or syllable is repeated several to many times and the flow of speech is interrupted.

Propulsion: Disturbance of gait typical of parkinsonism in which the patient, during walking, steps faster and faster with progressively shorter steps and passes from a walking to a running pace and may fall forward.

Rigidity: Refers in medical usage to a type of muscular stiffness encountered when examining Parkinson patients. It is characterized by a constant, even resistance to passive manipulation of the limbs. It is due to a failure of reciprocal relaxation of the antagonist muscles.

Retropulsion: Involuntary stepping backward; the reverse of propulsion.

Striatum: Short for corpus striatum (see above).

Substantia nigra: Anatomical term (from Latin, meaning black substance) referring to darkly pigmented area in the upper brainstem that can be seen on visual inspection of specimens of human and primate brains. Substantia nigra cells contain both pigment granules and large amounts of dopamine.

Sleeping sickness: Popular term used during the 1920s and 1930s to refer to encephalitis lethargica. (There is another, more commonly known disease limited to Central Africa caused by a parasite transmitted to man and cattle by the bite of the tsetse fly that is also called sleeping sickness.)

Seborrhea: Increased discharge of the oily secretion sebum from the sebaceous glands of the skin.

Seborrheic dermatitis: Inflammation of the skin sometimes associated with seborrhea.

Solanaceous alkaloids: Bitter tasting alkaline substances extracted from plants of the family Solanaceae and including the botanical drugs atropine, scopolamine, and hyoscyamine.

Stereotactic surgery: Surgical technique for operating deep in the brain without direct visualization and without opening the brain; a long needle-like instrument attached to a frame bolted temporarily to the skull is passed into the brain at angles calculated from anatomical landmarks to bring it to a predetermined target. This technique makes it possible to produce very small lesions deep in the brain with considerable precision and minimal injury to the brain.

Shaking palsy: Old popular term which James Parkinson employed to designate the specific disorder we now call Parkinson's disease.

Tremor: A regular rhythmic to-and-fro involuntary movement of small amplitude affecting a limb, the head, or the entire body.

Thalamotomy: Operation in which a small region of the thalamus is destroyed, usually done by stereotactic technique. Tremor and rigidity in parkinsonism and other conditions can be relieved by thalamotomy.

Thalamus: Anatomical term designating a mass of gray matter centrally placed deep in the brain near its base and serving as a major relay station for impulses traveling from the spinal cord and cerebellum to the cerebral cortex.

Tryptophan: One of the eight "essential" amino acids necessary for human nutrition; it is also the metabolic precursor of serotonin, an important chemical messenger in the corpus striatum.

Tyrosine: An amino acid occurring in nature and a normal component of the diet. It is a normal precursor in the synthesis of dopamine and adrenalin.

Vomiting center: Anatomical and physiological term referring to an area of the medulla oblongata in which are located several clusters of nerve cells that act to initiate and coordinate the act of vomiting to expel toxic substances from the stomach.

Von Economo's encephalitis: Another name for encephalitis lethargica (see above) honoring the Viennese neurologist Constantin von Economo who was given credit for first recognizing and describing the disorder.

Subject Index

SINEMET®
(Carbidopa-Levodopa, MSD)

alone, patients should be monitored closely during the dose adjustment period. Specifically, involuntary movements will occur more rapidly with SINEMET than with levodopa. The occurrence of involuntary movements may require dosage reduction.

Blepharospasm may be a useful early sign of excess dosage in some patients.

Current evidence indicates that other standard drugs for Parkinson's disease (except levodopa) may be continued while SINEMET is being administered, although their dosage may have to be adjusted.

If general anethesia is required, SINEMET may be continued as long as the patient is permitted to take fluids and medication by mouth. If therapy is interrupted temporarily, the usual daily dosage may be administered as soon as the patient is able to

SINEMET®
(Carbidopa-Levodopa, MSD)

take oral medication.

OVERDOSAGE

Management of acute overdosage with SINEMET is basically the same as management of acute overdosage with levodopa; however, pyridoxine is not effective in reversing the actions of SINEMET.

General supportive measures should be employed, along with immediate gastric lavage. Intravenous fluids should be administered judiciously and an adequate airway maintained. Electrocardiographic monitoring should be instituted and the patient carefully observed for the development of arrthythmias; if required, appropriate antiarrhythmic therapy should be given. The possibility that the patient may have taken other drugs as well as SINEMET should be taken into consideration. To date, no experience has been reported with dialysis; hence, its value in overdosage is not known.

SINEMET®
(Carbidopa-Levodopa, MSD)

HOW SUPPLIED

Tablets SINEMET 25-100 are yellow, oval, scored tablets, coded MSD 650. They are supplied as follows:
    NDC 0006-0650-68 bottles of 100
    NDC 0006-0650-28 unit dose packages of 100.
Tablets SINEMET 10-100 are dark dappleblue, oval, scored, uncoated tablets, coded MSD 647.
They are supplied as follows:
    NDC 0006-0647-68 bottles of 100
    NDC 0006-0647-28 unit dose packages of 100.
Tablets SINEMET 25-250 are light dappleblue, oval, scored, uncoated tablets, coded MSD 654. They are supplied as follows:
    NDC 0006-0654-68 bottles of 100
    NDC 0006-0654-28 unit dose packages of 100.

Storage
    Tablets SINEMET 10-100 and Tablets SINEMET 25-250 must be protected from light.

Manufactured by
MERCK SHARP & DOHME
DIV OF MERCK & CO., INC.,
WEST POINT, PA 19486, USA

TABLETS
SINEMET®
(CARBIDOPA-LEVODOPA, MSD)

DESCRIPTION

When SINEMET® (Carbidopa-Levodopa, MSD) is to be given to patients who are being treated with levodopa, levodopa must be discontinued at least eight hours before therapy with SINEMET is started. In order to reduce adverse reactions, it is necessary to individualize therapy. See the WARNINGS and DOSAGE AND ADMINISTRATION sections before initiating therapy.

Carbidopa, an inhibitor of aromatic amino acid decarboxylation, is a white, crystalline compound, slightly soluble in water, with a molecular weight of 244.3. It is designated chemically as (—)-L-α- hydrazino-α-methyl-β-(3,4-dihydroxybenzene) propanoic acid monohydrate, and has the following structural formula:

$$HO-C_6H_3(OH)-CH_2C(CH_3)COOH \cdot H_2O$$
$$|$$
$$NHNH_2$$

Tablet content is expressed in terms of anhydrous carbidopa which has a molecular weight of 226.3.

Levodopa, an aromatic amino acid, is a white, crystalline compound, slightly soluble in water, with a molecular weight of 197.2. It is designated chemically as (—)-L-α-amino-β (3,4-dihydroxybenzene) propanoic acid, and has the following structural formula:

$$HO-C_6H_3(OH)-CH_2CHCOOH$$
$$|$$
$$NH_2$$

SINEMET is supplied as tablets in three strengths:

SINEMET 25-100, containing 25 mg of carbidopa and 100 mg of levodopa.

SINEMET 10-100, containing 10 mg of carbidopa and 100 mg of levodopa.

SINEMET 25-250, containing 25 mg of carbidopa and 250 mg of levodopa.

Inactive ingredients are cellulose,

SINEMET®
(Carbidopa-Levodopa, MSD)

magnesium stearate, and starch. Tablets SINEMET 10-100 and 25-250 also contain FD&C Blue 2. Tablets SINEMET 25-100 also contain D&C Yellow 10 and FD&C Yellow 6.

ACTIONS

Current evidence indicates that symptoms of Parkinson's disease are related to depletion of dopamine in the corpus striatum. Administration of dopamine is ineffective in the treatment of Parkinson's disease apparently because it does not cross the blood - brain barrier. However, levodopa, the metabolic precursor of dopamine, does cross the blood-brain barrier, and presumably is converted to dopamine in the basal ganglia. This is thought to be the mechanism whereby levodopa relieves symptoms of Parkinson's disease.

When levodopa is administered orally it is rapidly converted to dopamine in extracerebral tissues so that only a small portion of a given dose is transported unchanged to the central nervous system. For this reason, large doses of levodopa are required for adequate therapeutic effect and these may often be attended by nausea and other adverse reactions, some of which are attributable to dopamine formed in extracerebral tissues.

Since levodopa competes with certain amino acids, the absorption of levodopa may be impaired in some patients on a high protein diet.

Carbidopa inhibits decarboxylation of peripheral levodopa. It does not cross the blood-brain barrier and does not affect the metabolism of levodopa within the central nervous system.

Since its decarboxylase inhibiting activity is limited to extracerebral tissues, administration of carbidopa with levodopa makes more levodopa available for transport to the brain. In dogs, reduced formation of dopamine in extracerebral tissues, such as the heart, provides protection against the development of dopamine-induced cardiac arrhythmias. Clinical studies tend to support the hypothesis of a similar protective effect in humans although controlled data are too limited at the present time to draw firm conclusions.

Carbidopa reduces the amount of levodopa required by about 75 percent and, when administered with levodopa, increases both plasma levels and the plasma half-life of levodopa, and decreases plasma and urinary dopamine and homovanillic acid.

In clinical pharmacologic studies, simultaneous administration of carbidopa and levodopa produced greater urinary excretion of levodopa in proportion to the excretion of dopamine than administration of the two drugs at separate times.

Pyridoxine hydrochloride (vitamin B_6), in oral doses of 10 mg to 25 mg. may reverse the effects of levodopa by increasing the rate of aromatic amino acid decarboxylation. Carbidopa inhibits this action of pyridoxine.

INDICATIONS

SINEMET is indicated in the treatment of the symptoms of idiopathic Parkinson's disease (paralysis agitans), post-encephalitic parkinsonism, and symptomatic parkinsonism which may follow injury to the nervous system by carbon monoxide intoxication and manganese intoxication. SINEMET is indicated in these conditions to permit the administration of lower doses of levodopa with reduced nausea and vomiting, with more rapid dosage titration, with a somewhat smoother response, and with supplemental pyridoxine (vitamin B_6).

The incidence of levodopa-induced nausea and vomiting is less with SINEMET than with levodopa. In many patients this reduction in nausea and vomiting will permit more rapid dosage titration.

In some patients a somewhat smoother antiparkinsonian effect results from therapy with SINEMET than with levodopa. However, patients with markedly irregular ("on-off") responses to levodopa have not been shown to benefit from SINEMET.

Since carbidopa prevents the reversal of levodopa effects caused by pyridoxine, SINEMET can be given to patients receiving supplemental pyridoxine (vitamin B_6).

Although the administration of carbidopa permits control of parkinsonism and Parkinson's disease with much lower doses of levodopa, there is no